Cancer Care in the Post-COVID World

Mark Foulkes • Helen Roe
Andreas Charalambous
Editors

Cancer Care in the Post-COVID World

A UK and European Perspective on Learning from the Pandemic

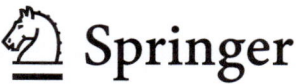

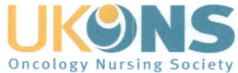

Editors
Mark Foulkes
Macmillan Lead Cancer Nurse and Nurse Consultant
Royal Berkshire NHS Foundation Trust
Reading, UK

Prof Andreas Charalambous PhD, MSc, BSc ⓘ
Department of Nursing Science
Cyprus University of Technology
Limassol, Cyprus

Helen Roe
Northern Centre for Cancer Care (Cumbria) (up to Dec 2022)
Newcastle upon Tyne Hospitals NHS Foundation Trust
Carlisle, UK

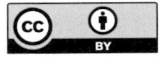

ISBN 978-3-031-33854-0   ISBN 978-3-031-33855-7 (eBook)
https://doi.org/10.1007/978-3-031-33855-7

© The Editor(s) (if applicable) and The Author(s) 2026. This book is an open access publication.

Open Access This book is licensed under the terms of the Creative Commons Attribution 4.0 International License (http://creativecommons.org/licenses/by/4.0/), which permits use, sharing, adaptation, distribution and reproduction in any medium or format, as long as you give appropriate credit to the original author(s) and the source, provide a link to the Creative Commons license and indicate if changes were made.

The images or other third party material in this book are included in the book's Creative Commons license, unless indicated otherwise in a credit line to the material. If material is not included in the book's Creative Commons license and your intended use is not permitted by statutory regulation or exceeds the permitted use, you will need to obtain permission directly from the copyright holder.

The use of general descriptive names, registered names, trademarks, service marks, etc. in this publication does not imply, even in the absence of a specific statement, that such names are exempt from the relevant protective laws and regulations and therefore free for general use.

The publisher, the authors and the editors are safe to assume that the advice and information in this book are believed to be true and accurate at the date of publication. Neither the publisher nor the authors or the editors give a warranty, expressed or implied, with respect to the material contained herein or for any errors or omissions that may have been made. The publisher remains neutral with regard to jurisdictional claims in published maps and institutional affiliations.

This Springer imprint is published by the registered company Springer Nature Switzerland AG
The registered company address is: Gewerbestrasse 11, 6330 Cham, Switzerland

If disposing of this product, please recycle the paper.

Introduction

The Covid-19 pandemic represented the most significant public health emergency of international concern (PHEIC) of the last 100 years. It resulted in global disruption, socio-economic upheaval on a huge scale and, sadly, a massive loss of life.
Infection with the SARS-CoV-2 virus disproportionally affected vulnerable populations, including older adults, women, lower-income communities, racial and ethnic minorities and individuals with underlying health conditions [1]. The final grouping of this list included people with a level of immunocompromise, such as individuals with a cancer diagnosis. This book addresses the effects of the Covid-19 pandemic upon this patient group, from a United Kingdom and European perspective and those who treated, cared and supported them throughout.

This book discusses the experience of patients with a cancer diagnosis and possibly receiving immunocompromising treatments. It also considers the impact on the health systems caring for these individuals whether from a perspective of patient management or flow to the effects on the education of healthcare workers during the pandemic.

The COVID-19 pandemic caused disruption but also provided a fertile opportunity for innovations in cancer care with an increased use of technology, treatment adaptation and rapid learning on the physiological impact of the SARS-CoV-2 virus on the cancer population and how they might be protected. This book considers these innovations and attempts to contextualise the learning from this period from a point of view of longer-term cancer care. There is also a consideration of the effectiveness of managing an unprecedented health crisis, the contribution of those working in cancer care and what was learned from their experiences.

An obvious consequence of the COVID-19 pandemic was the fear of illness and death, increased social isolation and the profound effect on the mental health of global populations. This effect was magnified in the population of persons diagnosed with cancer and healthcare providers across Europe and the United Kingdom. These effects and possible support mechanisms are considered in this book as well as any longer-term learning on the best way to maintain the mental health of health workers in cancer care and others supporting patients such as those working within the 'third sector'.

As we pass the 5-year anniversary of the commencement of the pandemic this book provides an opportunity to examine the immediate and longer-term effects of the COVID-19 pandemic on cancer care, to reflect on experiences and learning and to help us in developing and implementing potential strategies to integrate future resilience into cancer care. These will include the need for increased mental health support for both patients and oncology professionals, fostering an innovative approach to rapid learning and public health management and putting plans in place to mitigate the effects on cancer care of future pandemics.

Mark Foulkes
Helen Roe
Andreas Charalambous

Reference

1. Liu E, Dean CA, Elder KT (2023) The impact of COVID-19 on vulnerable populations. Front Publ Health 11:1267723

Contents

1	**Personal Experiences of Receiving Systemic Anti-cancer Treatment During the COVID -19 Pandemic** .... Helen Roe	1
2	**Research Background COVID and Cancer** .... Joanne Bird	17
3	**Haematological Perspectives on COVID-19 and Cancer** .... Karen Sayal	29
4	**Telehealth, Digital Technology and the COVID-19 Pandemic, the Impact on Cancer Care** .... Mark Foulkes	39
5	**Virtual Consultations: Considering Staff Training and Patient Experience** .... Catherine Oakley and Emma Rowland	53
6	**European Perspectives on Cancer and the Pandemic** .... Constantina Cloconi, Christina Alexopoulou, Nicole Zamba, Mary Economou, and Andreas Charalambous	61
7	**The Effect of the COVID-19 Pandemic on the Charity Sector** .... Dany Bell	73
8	**Impact on Cancer Education COVID-19** .... Karen Campbell	87
9	**The Psychological Impact of COVID-19 on Healthcare Staff: Support Mechanisms and Leadership Approaches** .... Lucy Grant and Mark Foulkes	97
10	**Guilt and Miracles: A Personal History of the Nightingale Hospital** .... Eamonn Sullivan	109

11	**Cancer Patient Management and Flow During the COVID-19 Pandemic** 125
	Mark Foulkes
12	**The Delivery of Systemic Anti-Cancer Therapies (SACT) During the COVID-19 Pandemic.**............................... 141
	Mark Foulkes
13	**The Legacy of the COVID-19 Pandemic in Cancer Care** 151
	Helen Roe

Personal Experiences of Receiving Systemic Anti-Cancer Treatment During the COVID-19 Pandemic

Helen Roe

Check Your Experience
1. If you work in healthcare, consider the changes in care delivery which took place during the COVID-19 pandemic which might have impacted patients directly.
2. Consider the impact of becoming isolated, losing most face-to-face contact with family members and professionals when you are most vulnerable from the treatment you are receiving and a pandemic we knew very little about.

Introduction

With the emergence of the coronavirus SARS-CoV-2 (COVID-19) pandemic in 2020 [1], lives were changed instantly due to the potential impact this virus would have.

Professionals working in healthcare implemented changes, almost overnight, to continue the delivery of care. There was a need to focus on the safety of both patients and professionals in terms of minimising possible exposure to the virus. The ongoing care for patients with cancer needed to consider the potential impact of the virus with the known consequences of having a cancer diagnosis and receiving potentially immunosuppressive treatment.

Given the short time frame to make changes, the normal processes for implementing any changes were not in place. Instead, changes were made and reviewed as more data became available regarding the impact of the virus on the general public and patients with cancer. Many of the changes involved patients attending clinical areas less and being reviewed in a virtual setting.

The need to support patients and their loved ones was greater than ever due to the number of questions regarding a poorly understood virus. Concerns included

H. Roe (✉)
Northern Centre for Cancer Care (Cumbria) (up to Dec 2022),
Newcastle upon Tyne Hospitals NHS, Foundation Trust, Carlisle, UK

© The Author(s) 2026
M. Foulkes et al. (eds.), *Cancer Care in the Post-COVID World*,
https://doi.org/10.1007/978-3-031-33855-7_1

conceivable consequences for them in terms of their treatment and potential impact on their clinical outcomes. At a time when their demand for support and monitoring was increased, the pandemic left them more isolated. Healthcare professionals needed to utilise any available evidence or ideas to develop new ways of working to provide treatment and undertake evaluation of responses and toxicities.

A key change was the way communication occurred between patients and professionals in a safe and timely manner. This involved a greater use of technology, a concept not all patients or professionals were necessarily familiar with. There needed to be a continuous balancing of the potential benefits of a patient receiving SACT against the equally potential consequences of the virus.

A group of patients have shared glimpses into how their lives were changed during the pandemic to assist professionals in gaining a better understanding of living with a cancer diagnosis, receiving SACT and importantly how their lives were changed overnight by the emergence of the SARS-CoV-2 virus. This information will hopefully assist with reflection and offer future considerations when implementing changes, potentially in response to other health crises.

Cancer Diagnosis

Macmillan Cancer Support has described the overwhelming impact which a cancer diagnosis can have on an individual, their family and friends and how some can be left feeling frightened and unsure of how to manage their future. Many individuals consider the impact a cancer diagnosis will have on their everyday life in terms of possible loss of independence, possible change of lifestyle, being treated differently by others and needing to rely on someone else. Other considerations are related to how a cancer diagnosis may affect their job and importantly the possible financial implications, along with the possible need to take time off work to attend appointments, etc. Individuals often discuss concerns regarding their long-term survival and ultimately whether they will die due to the cancer diagnosis [2].

Understandably all these changes to a person's life can leave them with many mixed emotions and mood changes, some they have not previously experienced. These emotions may include fear and anxiety around handing over control of their body, a loss of control of their life, concerns around their possible treatment options, worries around if the treatment will work and, if not, what happens then. There is a potential psychological impact on them as a person and those around them; they may experience sadness and/or anxiety regarding the above and possible depression. A cancer diagnosis may be only one aspect a person is facing, i.e. health concerns or other issues impacting their life, for example, difficulties with their finances. A cancer diagnosis can often leave a person feeling alone and isolated, not wishing to burden others with their concerns.

A cancer diagnosis may come with physical consequences relating to the site of the cancer and caused by required treatments such as surgery, radiotherapy or SACT/chemotherapy and their possible side effects, i.e. fatigue, pain or altered body image. These not only occur at the point of diagnosis but throughout the person's future life, potentially having a significant impact on their well-being and quality of life in terms of physical, psychological, social and spiritual aspects.

Some describe life after a cancer diagnosis as an 'emotional rollercoaster', never knowing what the next day may bring or if they will have the emotional and physical energy to deal with events. One continual concern felt by many, although often not explicitly spoken about is the fear of recurrence [3].

P1 *Thinking back to when I first received my cancer diagnosis, I was shocked even though I hadn't been 100% for a while beforehand and blamed everything but my health. After being told I had cancer my main concern was would I die and if so, how long would I have? Shortly followed by concerns for my family who would watch me go through treatment and its side-effects. I would never be 'me' again – I would be someone with cancer and I probably would lose my hair, and everyone would then know I had cancer. On that day I thought my life was over, however since then the cancer keeps coming back and has never gone away (palliative), but I am still here 15 years later.*

P3 *I'm not really sure I can remember much about my initial diagnosis and the conversation with the doctor, except for the word CANCER. I can however remember being told the cancer had returned and could no longer be cured. Over recent years and during the pandemic these conversations continued. I'm just so glad it has been the same nurse explaining this to me and my husband each time rather than a stranger. She knows us and also how to pitch the information that is right for us.*

P5 *My initial diagnosis was following a routine mammogram, I was not only told I had cancer but that it had spread and could not be cured – all in one conversation. I just remember looking at my partners face as this news changed everyone around me's life too, we would never be 'us' again. I really struggle some days and wonder why I'm putting myself through this, but then I think of my family and what they mean to me.*

Emergence of the Coronavirus SARS-CoV-2

The end of January 2020 saw the first case of severe acute respiratory syndrome coronavirus 2 (SARS-CoV-2) in the United Kingdom, a condition which later on 11/02/2020 was named COVID-19. Only a few weeks after first being detected in the United Kingdom, the first death was reported in March 2020 [4].

As a result of the spread and potential impact on life of this virus, the UK government was required to take urgent action in an attempt to minimise suffering and save lives [2, 3]. Across the United Kingdom, this involved the introduction of regular televised update briefings by the government to provide information to the general public, which very soon became part of everyday living. In the middle of March 2020, the Prime Minister explained how he believed, based on available evidence, that with simple steps like staying at home for 14 days if you had a cough or a fever, we would be able to turn the tide in around 12 weeks [5].

However, a week later saw more stringent measures being introduced, which impacted everyone's 'normal' lives. One of the primary focuses at that time was to attempt to protect the National Health Service (NHS) from becoming overwhelmed. These measures included:

- Staying at home
- Not meeting people you did not live with
- Utilising food delivery services
- Travel only when absolutely necessary, i.e. medical needs
- One form of daily exercise (outside the home)

The 26th of March 2020 saw an event that many had not expected nor seen anything similar to in their lifetime—the country was placed in 'lockdown' after the Coronavirus Act 2020 received Royal Assent [6,7]. This resulted in the introduction of more rigid measures with possible penalties and included:

- Social distancing
- Stopping non-essential contact with others
- Stopping unnecessary travel
- Working from home whenever possible
- Only leaving the home for one episode of socially distanced exercise
- Avoiding public areas
- Only using the NHS when essential
- People with some health conditions were required to 'shield' for 12 weeks, which included a cancer diagnosis

P3 *All of a sudden, I became known as 'high risk' and 'vulnerable', these were words I had NEVER associated with me, even though I had incurable breast cancer.*

P4 *The psychological impact of not being able to give kisses and cuddles from a parent to a child as would have previously been considered totally natural, greatly impacted on our family life and continues to do so now as so many people are still contracting COVID.*

Life Changed

From that point on, the COVID pandemic and the accompanying restrictions had varying degrees of impact on a person's everyday life due to the need for social distancing and the wearing of face coverings. Some people were furloughed (temporarily paused) from work or needed to work from home and not mix with others. These imposed changes were often referred to by many as living in a 'bubble'. There were consequences for vital organisations as well as individuals, i.e. the closure of schools often led to children missing lessons and exams as they frequently needed to be home-schooled. During the COVID-19 pandemic, there were a number of separate lockdowns, dependent on available data and incidence rates which resulted in daily lives needing to be performed in a virtual world, for example, communication via video links, online shopping and tutoring. The initial uncertainties regarding the pandemic and how long it may last led to panic buying and rationing of essential food items as well as do-it-yourself (DIY) items as people turned to home improvements and gardening.

Within the United Kingdom, regarding lockdowns and restrictions, there was an added difficulty in that all four nations had slightly different restriction requirements and there were also area variations dependent on the incidence rate. This caused difficulties for people commuting over borders for work or healthcare, something which may have impacted other countries too. Restrictions in other countries also needed to be considered, even when UK lockdowns were eased in terms of travel between countries.

Once testing became established later in the COVID-19 pandemic, everyone needed to monitor their own symptoms and decide if they were required to undertake a test to establish if they were COVID-positive and therefore would have needed to self-isolate. Cancer patients receiving chemotherapy/SACT were familiar with monitoring their temperature and their cancer or treatment-related symptoms. However, along with the general public, they quickly learnt to undertake both lateral flow tests (LFTs) and polymerase chain reaction (PCR) tests and knew who to contact if concerned, along with taking required action if they had tested positive. In the United Kingdom, everyone was encouraged to have the NHS COVID and 'Track and Trace' applications on their mobile telephone to monitor any contacts they might have inadvertently had over time with a possible positive case.

P1 *The pandemic restrictions were so hard – although I had metastatic breast cancer, I had been stable for a while and didn't get many side effects from my treatment and so my life had been fairly normal. Now I couldn't meet friends for a coffee and a chat (support), couldn't wonder around the shops, everything was now online. Even walking the dog was stressful, in case anyone came near us, major panic if they started to speak to me. Living in a 'family bubble' definitely tested all of our patience.*

P2 *Life really changed beyond belief during the pandemic – social distancing, wearing face coverings, not hugging each other, thinking everyone you meet might have COVID, especially if they cough! Who would ever have thought we would all have a Christmas family lunch by video link, it stopped the family arguments about who's turn it was to cook.*

P6 *We had to do the food shopping on line, lots of things we wanted were no longer available or we were limited to how many we could have, things like anti-bacterial wipes, toilet rolls, pasta and long-life milk became luxuries. Everything was delivered to the garage, stayed there for 24 hours then all the packaging was cleaned, and things came into the house. The highlight of the day would be to see what 'substitutes' we had received!*

Cancer and the COVID Pandemic

Prior to the pandemic, patients with a cancer diagnosis often felt isolated due to their diagnosis and possible treatment; however, the COVID pandemic brought them added concerns as they were categorised as being high risk if they contracted COVID, and as such, their preventative measures became even more stringent than for the general public. They were classed as high risk due to their diagnosis of cancer and the treatment they were receiving, along with possible toxicities and the treatment being potentially immunosuppressive [8]. Other key factors regarding their individual risk were their possible comorbidities and for some being advanced in age [9].

Patients and their families were also worried regarding what might happen if they contracted COVID, such as concerns around their treatment being delayed leading to a cancer recurrence or progression. If they attended appointments at the hospital, they may have put themselves at greater risk of contracting COVID, but if they stayed away, a change with their cancer may have been missed. [8]

As the required lockdown measures included healthcare, patients found themselves in an environment where traditional healthcare no longer existed, leaving many feeling isolated and disconnected, leading to some experiencing a negative impact on their mental, emotional and physical health [10]. The consequences of the pandemic also posed many financial implications for patients and their families in terms of income and employment with many family members feeling guilty [8, 11].

Communication between the patient and healthcare professionals also changed [11], with face-to-face consultations stopping immediately unless necessary, for example, if information had to be discussed or if an individual patient had specific needs such as deafness or other communication difficulties and no alternative form of exchanging information could be found. Communication became virtual, that is, via telephone or video. Consideration was needed as to patient access to computer and adequate Internet connection, especially in rural areas. Some people had hardly or never previously used computers as a way to communicate virtually. A further consideration was the need for professionals to have adequate access to computers and appropriate services, especially as some were required to work from home. Lives definitely changed and the opportunity to observe nonverbal communication and facial expressions had been lost due to compulsory wearing of face coverings and visors. Listening for changes in a person's voice such as pauses was difficult to pick up during telephone conversations. Simple cues such as watching how a person walked into the room, sat down and engaged with their family and professionals had been lost. Relatives who previously played a key role in sharing communication or expressing the patients' concerns were missed as they may not have been in the patient's 'bubble'.

> P2 *At the beginning of the pandemic I think I was more afraid about COVID than I had been receiving my cancer diagnosis. I know my cancer team know about my cancer and its treatment, but none of us really know anything about COVID, how it might affect me and my fear was would I die of COVID rather than cancer.*

P4 *I became totally paranoid, probably made worse by me staying at home worrying about my family mixing with other people and then returning home. My husband's boss was not very understanding initially when he asked about changing his job slightly to help protect me. My cancer nurse wrote a letter explaining things and then he was much better. My husband and son had to strip off when entering the house, put their clothes in the washing machine and have a shower before doing anything. Don't think we had ever done so much washing.*

Patients became unsure of who to turn to for advice and often turned to social media and online support groups [10]. This enabled them to access general and specific information regarding the potential impact of the pandemic in general, but not related to them as an individual. Much of the information was produced by charities at short notice to meet an urgent need from patients and their relatives; one example was 'Coronavirus and cancer treatment' produced by Cancer Research UK [12]. The topic of how the pandemic impacted charities will be discussed further in Chap. 7.

Unrecognisable Healthcare

Given the speed of the spread of the pandemic throughout the world, immediate changes were required in healthcare; time for planning, monitoring, seeking approval and finally implementing change was not an option; pathways and processes were required to change overnight as existing operating policies were no longer fit for purpose [8, 9]. Changes were required to protect vulnerable patients and reduce the potential impact of COVID on their lives and treatment outcomes as much as possible. The focus was on maintaining services, ensuring the safety of both the patient and the professional, yet at the same time minimising hospital attendances to help prevent the service from becoming overwhelmed and unable to cope [13]. Another key focus had to be around protecting staff during the pandemic in order to be able to deliver the care patients required.

Given the above key considerations, reflecting on my own experience within the clinical area where I was employed during the pandemic and the women received their treatments, we all witnessed many changes. Our local treatment area changed from being one that many described as a clinical extension of their home where they came for treatment to an almost unwelcoming lonely place. Everything suddenly became sterile, and if it could not be wiped repeatedly, it was removed, and people's appointment times needed to be altered according to risk. Doors to treatment unit became locked, and doorbells were introduced. On arrival, people were asked key questions about their health, possible COVID-19 contacts they may have had and attendance elsewhere in the hospital as this excluded them (for a period of time) from entering the chemotherapy/SACT treatment units as they were classed as a potential risk [9]. After the questions came the temperature check and, at various times during the pandemic, a COVID test, all of which added to the degree of stress someone attending for treatment already experiences. To further add to their stress levels, they were required to receive their treatment unaccompanied, with no one to chat to, to offer them support and reassurance and to remind them of questions to ask, plus they were often in a room on their own [9].

Even when a person attended for their SACT, there was uncertainty if the drugs would have been available due to many shortages in the supply chain and if the appropriate staff were available to deliver the treatment [11] or might they have contracted COVID and be required to isolate at home. Very quickly following the start of the pandemic, we saw on the news that some treatment units closed for a few weeks, some drugs (in common with other items) were in short supply, people were fearful of attending healthcare settings, and waiting lists grew as healthcare attempted to deal with the influx of COVID-positive patients and their health needs. For example, in the United Kingdom, operating theatres became an extension of intensive care units, and staff were redeployed to areas of greatest needs, i.e. a chemotherapy nurse could find themselves working on surgical units or intensive care units.

Options that did not require the patient to attend the hospital were also explored at great speed including home delivery of medication via postal or courier services, and even drive-through pick-up points were established, often linked to local chemists or supermarkets [14]. Home administration of treatments by appropriately trained professionals, and in some cases, patients administering their own treatments was also utilized. This is discussed in greater detail in Chap. 11 regarding COVID-19 and SACT.

P1 *I have been attending for treatment on my own for years and at times it felt a bit like a social event, chatting to other people having treatment and in some cases offering reassurance to people just starting treatment. Now coming for my treatment was alien – the locked door, the doorbell, waiting for the door to be answered, the tests, the questions, nothing looked like before – all the walls were bare. Face coverings definitely ended any conversation, I just looked at people over my mask and wondered if they have or had 'it'.*

P2 *I just needed to get in and out as quick as possible. I would sit and watch the nurses going from patient to patient, trying to reassure us all. Listening to the phone and the doorbell constantly ringing. I did wonder what the pandemic meant to them and their families, possibly putting themselves at risk by caring for us. I thought about how hot they must be in all their protective clothing, but still they carried on caring for us all. One day I counted how many times one nurse washed her hands and then wondered what her skin must be like.*

P3 *The community nurse came to me house and took my bloods on the doorstep and then went down the road to the next patient. All my care continued on time whether at the hospital or at home – much easier and more efficient than trying to sort my supermarket delivery.*

P4 *It was bad enough being at home most of the time on my own worrying about what might happen to me, but to be dropped off at the door for my treatment was unbearable. One of the areas my cancer has spread to was to my brain and I couldn't always remember everything. The day before my treatment my husband*

and I wrote a list of questions and I asked the nurse to write the answers down for my husband to read later. The problems was when the nurse asked me a question and I sometimes got the answer wrong. We found a way around this in that when we had the pre-treatment chat my husband joined in on the mobile from the car.

Husband of P5 *Every time my wife attended the GP surgery to have her bloods checked or attended the hospital for any reason, I felt scared. I know these events were previously routine and part of our everyday life, but now was different. What if someone did have COVID (but didn't know) and they coughed, would the mask be sufficient? What if the chair* etc *hadn't been cleaned properly? I even worry if no-one answered the door and she couldn't get in for her treatment. I told myself I was being stupid but I was just so concerned and everything was out of my control.*

P6 *Very early on our nurse wrote to all of us and explained everything – continuing with treatment – although they may change slightly, how the unit would appear different, CT scans and heart scans would continue as close to normal timings as before, appointments would need to be video or telephone, face to face only if really necessary. The one thing she did that probably kept us all and our families sane was she created an email account for us all to contact her on with any questions (and there were many). She always replied – email, phone, appointment whatever was needed. Me and my family still use it now to let her know things and I hear others talking about it.*

Treatment Options

As professionals we needed to constantly consider the risk and benefit of someone receiving SACT during the pandemic or whether they were potentially being put at greater risk as a consequence of receiving treatment and its effect on their body, in particular their immunity [15]. With great speed several key expert groups came together and reviewed the limited available data regarding the potential impact of COVID on people with a cancer diagnosis and specifically for those receiving SACT [15, 16].

All patients needed to be individually assessed regarding possible risk/benefit in terms of receiving SACT during the pandemic [16]. This included considering:

- Tumour site
- Clinical setting, i.e. neoadjuvant, adjuvant or palliative.
- Co-morbidities
- Individual factors—age, sex and ethnicity
- Lines of treatment previously received
- Vaccination status—COVID
- Available data regarding potential impact of COVID

Only after considering the above and having a joint discussion with the patient could a shared decision be made [16].

As the potential impact of the pandemic on cancer care was unknown, difficult decisions needed to be made in terms of prioritising SACT for where the greatest benefit could be expected, i.e. neoadjuvant and adjuvant, ensuring that all comorbidities were considered, i.e. respiratory or cardiac conditions [17]. One option considered was to reduce the number of cycles of treatment or consider using endocrine options instead. Consideration needed to be given to the lines of palliative treatment someone may have received and the potential benefit they were likely to gain based on previous research and whether a treatment delay or omission would be a more appropriate choice based on the potential risks associated with potential COVID exposure [18, 19].

Later in the pandemic, risks to individuals were reduced by ensuring all patients were fully vaccinated for both COVID and influenza, as well as being tested for COVID pretreatment. The use of 24-hour helplines for those receiving treatments was reinforced, ensuring oncology input into the care and decision-making if a patient was admitted to a hospital. There was also a more widespread use of prophylactic granulocyte-colony-stimulating factor (GCSF) to minimise the risk of neutropenia during treatment [17]. A major concern which needed to be overcome was people's fear of attending hospitals, even when unwell, for fear of contracting COVID [19].

In England the National Cancer Drug Fund (CDF) offered more flexibility for treating patients receiving treatments funded by the CDF regarding continuing with treatment through the pandemic. For those already receiving a treatment, these were individually approved via the CDF until they, or their healthcare professional, jointly decided on stopping or switching treatment. This change meant there needed to be greater discussion regarding risk and benefit of receiving treatment with the patient, and the responsibility for any changes lies entirely with the prescribing professional. This heightened the need for clearly documented accounts of discussions that took place and clear justifications for any decisions made [15, 21].

For people with metastatic cancer receiving SACT, it was assumed based on the available evidence that this group would be more susceptible to developing severe infection and possible complications. For others receiving novel anticancer treatments (i.e. targeted therapies), the potential consequences were unknown [17, 19].

P2 *At the start of the pandemic I was already on my 4th line of palliative treatment, and I read on a patient forum about them stopping some treatments at this point due to the COVID risk. However, to me it would be stopping my lifeline as my treatment was keeping me alive.*

P3 *Throughout the pandemic all my scans carried on, although waiting for the results caused me more anxiety and sleepless nights, I can only imagine how unbearable I was waiting for results which took longer. I dreaded the news that the cancer had spread as I thought that would be the end of treatment and I would be left to die. That day never came as all my scans showed stable disease and I'm still on the same treatment – such a relieve.*

P5 *I heard lots of conversations about treatments being stopped or changed, risk of getting COVID, palliative patients being at greater risk patient, initial uncertainties around continuing to receive funded treatments – it was only happening to others so not a problem for me, but I still worried. But then my scan showed progression and my treatment needed to change – it was now 'real and scary' and happening to me. My nurse and I discussed my previous treatments, where the progression was, 'normal' next line of treatment options, COVID risk and impact on options. Then came the recommendation for me to receive a treatment option with one drug 'missing' – everything she spoke to me about made sense, but would it work or would the cancer carry on spreading? I went with the recommendation and had the same treatment throughout the pandemic until I had further progression recently and now I'm receiving a non-COVID (normal) treatment option.*

Clinical Research

Cancer clinical research was and remains a vital part of cancer care, with around one in six people actively taking part in research to either access new methods of care or newer treatment options or to influence future care delivery [20].

During the pandemic, almost all clinical trials in the UK were suspended [18], with new studies or the opening of new participation sites halted to focus on urgently needed research around COVID-19 [22]. This action had a negative impact on those who may have exhausted standard treatments and may be requiring treatment offer via studies [18]. This suspension also had a financial impact in terms of funding acquired from current research activity required to support future research opportunities [20]. This issue is discussed in detail in Chap. 2.

The design of existing studies that did continue during the pandemic required protocol amendments to minimise patients needing to attend hospitals where possible, i.e. home delivery of treatments [22]. Other key considerations were regarding obtaining consent and clinical reviews; again this was an area where telephone and video consultations were utilised similar to elsewhere in healthcare [23].

Many cancer research teams were redeployed to undertake SARS-CoV-2 research studies or to support front line staff caring for patients [20]. A change was also seen in the requirements for study activities previously provided in the hospital setting now being approved and provided by local and community settings in some countries to ensure vital research continued [23].

P2 *As patients we were all signing up for studies, but I had no idea that the nurses were also taking part in studies until a nurse mentioned it one day—they were undergoing twice week PCR tests, not just LFT test, they were having blood samples taken every other week at one point, filling in questionnaires. They were not only focusing on us but making a difference to everyone and I remember in one of the weekly Government briefing I heard them mention the study the nurses were taking part in.*

P5 *As the pandemic started, I was just about to start treatment as part of a study, but this was stopped—no idea how long for. After many discussions between my husband and I and my nurse, not to mention sleepless nights I started a 'traditional' treatment instead. Until my first CT scan I always thought if the cancer was worse COVID would be to blame, not the cancer.*

P6 *I had never been offered the opportunity to take part in any research studies, but during the pandemic I wanted to help. I signed up for many studies—COVID testing, blood samples, ones about my quality of life, any I could sign up for, after all I was only sat at home thinking.*

On-Treatment Reviews

A key requirement for patients during the pandemic was the provision of good information and support services regarding coping during the pandemic. This took the form of ongoing communication between the patient and the professional and information provided in written or video format to reinforce conversations that had occurred [8]. Virtual cancer care appointments were introduced across healthcare to minimise patient exposure to the hospital environment where possible [9]. Although the concept of telemedicine has been around for several years in other healthcare settings, few studies have assessed the patient satisfaction of this type of review in the cancer setting [24].

Any virtual reviews were considered safe and cost-effective; they were implemented virtually overnight as a way of monitoring patients during the pandemic whilst they continued to receive SACT. These reduced patients' need to attend clinical areas and lessened the possible risk of contracting COVID, especially as many treatments left them immunocompromised [24]. Although individuals, both general and those who contributed to this chapter, did not feel their care was unduly compromised by this method, they perceived the patient-professional interaction was not the same as personal face-to-face contact was missing [25]. Another consideration was trying to reduce the number of professional interactions a patient with cancer was required to have whilst receiving SACT and if these could be combined. [24]

Many healthcare professionals in the United Kingdom already had experience and qualifications in advanced communication skills; however, the requirements for a virtual consultation were very different from a face-to-face consultation, as all nonverbal cues were missing and the opportunity for physical examination if required was also missing [25]. In my own experience as a multiprofessional team, we had to work much closer as one team and rely on opinions of colleagues.

The ability and skills in accessing technology and the Internet for some receiving SACT were problematic, along with confidence in using it during virtual reviews, not to mention poor telephone networking or Internet access for many living in rural settings. Due to social distancing, many patients lost the support of a family member during the consultation, and virtual reviews offered an opportunity for a family member to be present [25].

Virtual consultations may be one COVID pandemic that required change to healthcare delivery that many patients have expressed a hope they continue after the pandemic. Reasons given by patients around this change related to removing the need for travel time, feeling safer in their own home and being at less risk of contracting possible infections [25]. Studies have shown that patients with breast cancer were satisfied with this form of communication and found it easy to navigate [24]. This is something that does appear to be continuing across healthcare in appropriate settings and with more clear methodology, for instance, alternating face-to-face and telephone reviews as the many COVID restrictions are reduced. Consideration was required in terms of possible compromise of the patient professional relationship and potential exclusion of those with poor access to, or difficulties with, technology and Internet connectivity [25]. Looking forward a potential adaptation would need to be around patient selection, for example, a patient established on treatment may find a virtual consultation works well for them in comparison to a new patient starting treatment who may have many questions, face uncertainties and would therefore benefit from a face-to-face consultation [24]. It seems certain that there will be many opportunities for evaluation in terms of patient and professional satisfaction. Clinical outcomes may be improved in some clinical situations where face-to-face reviews should definitely be fully re-implemented.

The topic of how the pandemic impacted the introduction of technology in healthcare and virtual consultations will be discussed further in Chap. 4.

P1 *I was well established on my current treatment and have been for quite a while – my scans and bloods stable and no real side effects. Having a telephone review in place of face-to-face visits worked well for me and meant I didn't need to keep going to the hospital. Also knowing I could email my nurse with any questions also worked well for me, I knew she was busy with other patients, but that she would reply.*

P2 *Telephone review worked most of the time for me, plus meant my husband could still be part of the discussion too. My treatment was put on hold at one point and I needed x-rays etc due to my symptoms as my nurse thought I may have picked up COVID – at this point I would have preferred a face to face consultation but I understood why this was not possible, instead she arranged a video review. I didn't have COVID and it was a side effect to my treatment - this made me realise how similar the symptoms could be and how careful I needed to be and how difficult things must be for the team looking after me.*

P3 *I never thought I would look forward to receiving a phone call from the hospital, but when my nurse rang, it was so reassuring to hear her voice, sometimes I could feel myself starting to cry when she said it was her. We discussed my treatment and any side effects, importantly she still had time to discuss everyday things and I felt she was interested in how I was managing and didn't merely focus on my cancer and treatment.*

P6 *I know I struggled with telephone consultations as I couldn't read my nurses facial expressions that told me more than words did. She understood this, also the fact I needed my husband to join in too (I have brain metastases) as I often forget things at times. When possible we did a video call or she would email me and my husband a summary of what we had spoken about – which I received the same day (much quicker than a hospital letter). When face to face consultation returned, I thought it would be much better, however the mask still hide the facial expressions, although I am now getting better at 'reading' people's eyes.*

Ongoing Impact of COVID

Patients continue to receive cancer treatments in the post-pandemic healthcare setting that has changed and is not likely to return to how they were delivered pre-pandemic. Even though most COVID control measures have now been removed, in most areas, individuals continued to be tested before starting treatments for many months and years, along with attending units that remained locked and accessible by ringing the bell.

All patients were encouraged to receive both COVID booster and flu vaccines and report when they felt unwell, even though they knew this could impact their treatment. COVID antiviral agents were introduced in the United Kingdom in 2021 and continued to offer some security to those high-risk patients who contract COVID [26], although the majority of patients with a solid tumour disease appeared to remain well and largely asymptomatic.

During the pandemic and given the documented higher mortality rates for patients with cancer, some patients tended to focus more on their illness and gave greater consideration regarding their possible mortality. For some this increased their anxiety levels and became a key consideration for professionals caring for patient receiving SACT, both during and following the pandemic in terms of required psychological support and surveillance [13].

The general population in the United Kingdom remains cautious in their lives, although they could go shopping, travel abroad, socialise again with non-family members or even hug one another, but remain aware that at any time another COVID variant or completely new pandemic may impact their lives and again alter the provision of healthcare.

Since the pandemic, all professionals continue to reflect on the impact of the pandemic and the rapidly implemented changes in the provision of care. We need to continually review the impact on individuals with cancer and importantly what can be learnt from them in order to shape the future of cancer care.

I wish to offer a much-needed thank you to the patients and their families for sharing their experiences of receiving systemic anti-cancer treatment during the pandemic.

Conflict of Interest The author does not have any conflict of interest to declare.

References

1. UK Health Security Agency (2022) Guidance – COVID-19: epidemiology, virology and clinical features (updated 17/05/2022). https://www.gov.uk/government/publications/wuhan-novel-coronavirus-background-information/wuhan-novel-coronavirus-epidemiology-virology-and-clinical-features. Accessed Mar 2023
2. Macmillan Cancer Support (2019) How are you feeling? The emotional effect of cancer. https://cdn.macmillan.org.uk/dfsmedia/1a6f23537f7f4519bb0cf14c45b2a529/769-source/mac11593e05nhow-are-you-feelinglowrespdf20190301. Accessed Mar 2023
3. Kállay É et al (2022) On top of that all, now COVID-19 too. A scoping review of specificities and correlates of fear of cancer recurrence in breast cancer patients during COVID-19. Breast 62:123–134. Accessed Mar 2023
4. Mahase E (2020) Covid-19: UK records first death, as world's cases exceed 1 000 000. Br Med J. https://www.bmj.com/content/368/bmj.m943. Accessed Mar 2023
5. Johnson B (2020) Prime Minister's statement on coronavirus (COVID-19): 16 March 2020. https://www.gov.uk/government/speeches/pm-statement-on-coronavirus-16-march-2020. Accessed Mar 2023
6. Johnson B (2020) Prime Minister's statement on coronavirus (COVID-19): 23 March 2020. https://www.gov.uk/government/speeches/pm-address-to-the-nation-on-coronavirus-23-march-2020. Accessed Mar 2023
7. UK Parliament (2020) Coronavirus Act. https://www.instituteforgovernment.org.uk/article/explainer/coronavirus-act-2020. Accessed Mar 2023
8. Kirby A et al (2022) Counting the social, psychological, and economic costs of COVID-19 for cancer patients. Support Care Cancer. https://doi.org/10.1007/s00520-022-07178-0. Accessed Mar 2023
9. Onestti C et al (2020) Oncology care organisation during COVID-19 outbreak. ESMO Open 5:e000853. https://doi.org/10.1136/esmoopen-2020-000853. Accessed Mar 2023
10. Moraliyage H et al (2021) Cancer in Lockdown: Impact of the COVID-19 pandemic on patients with cancer. Oncologist 26:E342–e344. Accessed Mar 2023
11. Dhada S et al (2021) Cancer Service during the COVID-19 pandemic: systematic review of patient's and caregiver's experiences. Cancer Manag Res 2021:13 5875-5887. Accessed Mar 2023
12. Cancer Research UK (2020) Coronavirus (COVID-19) and cancer treatment. https://www.cancerresearchuk.org/about-cancer/worried-about-cancer/coronavirus/cancer-treatment. Accessed Mar 2023
13. Sigorski D, Sobczuk P, Osmola M et al (2020) Impact of COVID-19 on anxiety levels amongst patients with cancer actively treated with systemic therapy. ESMO Open 5:e000970. https://doi.org/10.1136/esmoopen-2020-000970. Accessed Mar 2023
14. Cancer Research UK (2021) COVID innovations in cancer treatment. https://www.cancerresearchuk.org/sites/default/files/covid_innovations_-_treatment_1.pdf. Accessed Mar 2023
15. NHS (2021) NHS England interim treatment options during the COVID-19 pandemic. https://www.theacp.org.uk/userfiles/file/resources/covid_19_resources/nhs-england-interim-treatment-options-during-the-covid19-pandemic-pdf-8715724381-6-jan-2021.pdf. Accessed Mar 2023
16. National Institute for Health and Care Excellence (NICE) (2020) COVID-19 rapid guideline: delivery of systemic anticancer treatments. https://www.nice.org.uk/guidance/ng161/resources/covid19-rapid-guideline-delivery-of-systemic-anticancer-treatments-pdf-66141895710661. Accessed Mar 2023
17. El-Shakankery K, Kefas J, Crusz M (2020) Caring for our cancer patients in the wake of COVID-19. British J Cancer 123:4. https://doi.org/10.1038/s41416-020-0843-5. Accessed Mar 2023
18. Richards M et al (2020) The impact of the COVID-19 pandemic on cancer care. Nature Cancer 1:565–567. Accessed Mar 2023

19. Schrag D, Hershman D, Basch E (2020) Oncology practice during the COVID-19 pandemic. J Amer Med Assoc 323(20). https://doi.org/10.1001/jama.2020.6236. Accessed Mar 2023
20. Buckley-Mellor O (2020) What's happened to cancer clinical trials during the COVID-19 pandemic? https://news.cancerresearchuk.org/2020/11/04/whats-happened-to-cancer-clinical-trials-during-the-covid-19-pandemic/. Accessed Mar 2023
21. National Cancer Drug Fund (CDF) (2022) National Cancer Drugs Fund List V1.231 -Section C. Interim systemic anti-cancer therapy (SACT) treatment change options during the COVID-19 pandemic. https://www.england.nhs.uk/wp-content/uploads/2017/04/national-cdf-list-v1.231.pdf. Accessed Mar 2023
22. Thornton J (2020) Clinical trials suspended in UK to prioritise covid-19 studies and free up staff. British Med J 368:m1172. https://doi.org/10.1136/bmj.m1172. Accessed Mar 2023
23. Boughey J et al (2021) Impact of the COVID-19 pandemic on cancer clinical trials. Ann Surg Oncol 28(12):7311–7316. https://doi.org/10.1245/s10434-021-10406-2. Accessed Mar 2023
24. Johnson B et al (2021) The new normal? Patient satisfaction and usability of telemedicine in breast cancer care. Ann Surg Oncol 28:P5668–P5676. https://doi.org/10.1245/s10434-021-10448-6. Accessed Mar 2023
25. Hasson S et al (2021) Rapid implementation of telemedicine during the COVID-19 pandemic: Perspectives and preference of patients with cancer. Oncologist 26:e679–e685. Accessed Mar 2023
26. NHS (2022) Treatment for coronavirus (COVID-19). https://www.nhs.uk/conditions/coronavirus-covid-19/self-care-and-treatments-for-coronavirus/treatments-for-coronavirus/. Accessed Mar 2023

Open Access This chapter is licensed under the terms of the Creative Commons Attribution 4.0 International License (http://creativecommons.org/licenses/by/4.0/), which permits use, sharing, adaptation, distribution and reproduction in any medium or format, as long as you give appropriate credit to the original author(s) and the source, provide a link to the Creative Commons license and indicate if changes were made.

The images or other third party material in this chapter are included in the chapter's Creative Commons license, unless indicated otherwise in a credit line to the material. If material is not included in the chapter's Creative Commons license and your intended use is not permitted by statutory regulation or exceeds the permitted use, you will need to obtain permission directly from the copyright holder.

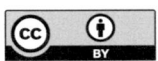

Research Background COVID and Cancer

2

Joanne Bird

Check Your Experience

If you work in research, how has your working day changed over the course of the COVID-19 pandemic?

If you do not routinely work in research, how did the pandemic change your view of clinical research?

What systems have been employed in your locality during the pandemic to continue to deliver cancer research?

What was the experience of cancer research patients in your clinical area? If you don't work in clinical research, talk to your local team.

Introduction

The COVID-19 pandemic had a profound and lasting effect on research, including cancer research across Europe. As the first wave began to spread across Europe, pictures of overwhelmed intensive care units were seen on all news channels and social media. Colleagues from Italy, one of the hardest hit countries early on, warned others of what was to come. The priority was to maintain clinical services, particularly intensive care services, and save lives by limiting the spread of SARS-CoV-2. Public isolation measures were introduced throughout the continent. The effect on cancer research came about through a number of changes:

1. Prioritisation of healthcare services
2. Prioritisation of SARS-CoV-2 research
3. Safety concerns
4. The economic impact on cancer research

J. Bird (✉)
Sheffield Teaching Hospitals NHS FT & University of Sheffield, Sheffield, South Yorkshire, UK
e-mail: Joanne.bird@sheffield.ac.uk

Stopping cancer research activity at the outbreak of the pandemic was much easier than trying to resume activity, particularly as infection levels rose and fell in subsequent waves. But while there have been challenges to the delivery of cancer research, there have been opportunities for innovation.

The interaction between SARS-CoV-2 and cancer, and subsequently SARS-CoV-2 vaccines and cancer, has become the focus of new research, in some instances giving rise to new innovation. As the virus has become endemic in the population of Europe, even if patients are not known to have tested positive or had symptoms, it can be assumed that all patients have been exposed, and this may cloud symptom reporting in future studies during periods of high prevalence or for patients experiencing the long-term effects of SARS-CoV-2 infection.

The Effect of the COVID-19 Pandemic on Cancer Research Delivery

Prioritisation of Healthcare Services

Italy was the first country in Europe to experience large numbers of people infected with SARS-CoV-2, and at the start of 2020, as the rest of Europe became aware of how overwhelmed the Italian healthcare system had become (particularly intensive care units), other countries began to prepare for the same. Non-essential services including research were suspended to allow resources to be diverted elsewhere. 80% of breast oncologists in Italy reported a reduction or suspension of research activity [1]. Research staff were redeployed to cover frontline clinical work. This immediately reduced capacity to continue existing clinical research. Healthcare professionals working in academic or teaching roles returned to clinical duties, often in place of time that they would have spent on research. For those who did not return to clinical duties, they found themselves having to transfer face-to-face teaching into an online format, often working from home with limited resources and with fewer members of staff to support students.

For those who remained in clinical research, this meant an increased workload, which contributed to a reduction in patient recruitment and delays in data collection [2]. Clinical research staff were also faced with managing the anxiety of patients who were considered vulnerable and had to explain complex information that often changed on a daily basis. With a reduced cancer research workforce, new clinical trials could not commence, recruitment was paused and the safety of those on clinical trials was prioritised.

Other professional groups also changed their work focus. Scientists who would have routinely been working on cancer research studies volunteered to assist with SARS-CoV-2 testing or used their skills and expertise to develop treatments for the virus or understand its effect on people with cancer [3]. Administration and operational staff supported healthcare infrastructure where they could utilise their skills elsewhere [3].

These workforce changes were further compounded by absences from work due to confirmed, or suspected, SARS-CoV-2 infection, periods of mandated isolation, new social distancing rules, bereavement and burnout. As the pandemic progressed, 'Long COVID' caused further staff to take long periods of sick leave. Longer-term absences due to SARS-CoV-2 infection increased during periods of high infection rates resulting in the continued need to prioritise healthcare services. For those continuing or returning to work in research, this resulted in loss of productivity and extended time to complete research.

Procedures that would have required intensive care or theatre facilities, including cancer surgery and some treatments, were cancelled to prioritise the care of patients with SARS-CoV-2. This was partly caused by shortages of oxygen and personal protective equipment (PPE). Patient safety (as discussed later) was also a priority. Early phase trials requiring access to ITU in case of a severe adverse drug reaction could not continue, partially due to the lack of resources.

In prioritising services to cope with the pandemic, there was a resulting reduction in capacity to perform investigations. This was partly due to the need for patients with SARS-CoV-2 infection to receive essential investigations, but also the increased need for cleaning and decontamination between patients. Essential safety monitoring for patients on cancer treatments and clinical trials such as imaging and cardiac monitoring was reduced in already busy services. Any investigations required for clinical research, above standard clinical care, could not be performed. This resulted in delays to data collection or missing data [2].

The overall effect was an abrupt halt to cancer research across Europe, whether laboratory-based, translational, clinical trials or patient experience research, and a sharp decrease in the number of patients being enrolled on clinical trials was seen [4]. As many studies are conducted internationally, restarting cancer research was more difficult as differing sites were experiencing different waves of the pandemic and had differing restrictions in place.

Prioritisation of COVID-19 Research

Once governments and healthcare organisations realised the potential impact of the COVID-19 pandemic, resources were poured into research into SARS-CoV-2 infection, and international collaboration happened in a way never before seen. There were two priorities:

1. Treatment for people contracting SARS-CoV-2 and becoming acutely unwell
2. Vaccination to protect the general population from severe illness

Investigational treatments were identified and developed quicker than we have previously seen in clinical research. The genetic sequence of the changing SARS-CoV-2 virus was shared online for researchers across the world to use resulting in early diagnostic tests and the development of vaccines [5]. The efforts put into research related to SARS-CoV-2, however, came at the cost of other research, including cancer research. Throughout Europe a sharp decrease in cancer clinical trial enrolment and a shift to trials investigating SARS-CoV-2 infection were observed [4]. Many researchers therefore commenced research to assess the effect of the virus on cancer patients.

While the focus of research was treatment and vaccination, a much wider variety of SARS-CoV-2-related research commenced. This included studies into the prevalence of the virus in healthcare workers, the psychological impact on healthcare professionals, the impact of remote consultations on patients and carers and the experience of end-of-life care during the pandemic and the experience of grief. Unfortunately, the vast increase in clinical trials related to the COVID-19 pandemic conducted in a short time meant that a number of low-quality trials were conducted. There has been criticism that the methodological quality of many rapidly conducted trials was questionable, and others were too small scale to provide conclusive results [6].

The need for the quick delivery of treatment for SARS-CoV-2 infection and vaccination trials meant that a large number of research staff were needed. Those with the appropriate knowledge and training were then diverted to delivering this essential work. Even large international trials were delivered at a rate never seen before. Technology facilitated international collaboration, but this research was only possible because of the skill and dedication of the clinical trials staff including clinical research nurses, data managers and other research staff who had the ability to adapt their skill set to the new environment. This demonstrated the importance of maintaining and nurturing this part of the workforce, whose skill set should not be underestimated.

The large number of pandemic-related research studies requiring regulatory approval had a further effect on cancer research. In the field of research regulation, SARS-CoV-2 studies were prioritised. This again resulted in the diversion of resources from other areas, including cancer. Even as services slowly restarted, SARS-CoV-2 studies were prioritised creating a backlog of other studies requiring approvals. Research not approved prior to the pandemic or requiring approval for a subsequent amendment had to wait, and doubtless, some studies never started. However, the speed at which pandemic studies passed through approval processes was unprecedented. Timescales that were usually months to years became days to weeks. The RECOVERY trial (an international multicentre randomised control trial with an adaptive platform design to identify treatments that may be beneficial for people hospitalised with suspected or confirmed COVID-19), for example, received approval within 4 days, and the first patient was enrolled 9 days after the protocol was finalised [7]. This could only be done with the drive and resources available during the pandemic and brings into question how a similar approach can be implemented to help cancer research recover and develop in the years to come.

Qualitative research was generally seen as a lower priority during a time of emergency, so it was stopped to prioritise other research where required. Where researchers were able to continue recruitment and data collection, methods needed to change to avoid face-to-face interactions. This meant that a swathe of online research was conducted via online surveys and telephone or video interviews. New research focused on experiences during the pandemic also took place online. This limited the pool of participants to those able to use online methods though more of the population became familiar with Internet-based technology out of necessity. Online methods enabled participation from a wider geographical area with limited costs whereby studies that would have been limited to the local population using face-to-face methods subsequently opened up to national or international recruitment. Participants could be interviewed across the world without participants or researchers having to leave their home. The UK Oncology Nursing Society experienced a sharp rise in requests to share survey requests via their newsletter, website and Twitter. The number of requests reduced from 2021 onwards, but a trend towards online research methods has been maintained.

Within the broad spectrum of cancer research, there is always a steady stream of masters and doctoral students contributing to every aspect of cancer care, whether laboratory, clinical, translational, educational, economic, epidemiologic or others. These are often conducted within tight timelines, sometimes with set timeframes for data collection, and longer studies are carefully planned. The pandemic left many students unable to collect data as planned, with suboptimal sample sizes or having to make major changes to their research plan. For a few years, there will be the regular appearance of a section or chapter reflecting on the effect of the pandemic on student research. Research-based qualifications can be stressful in more normal times, so the added personal and professional pressures of the pandemic will have affected many students, and there is no doubt that some promising careers will have been adversely altered. There will also be a wave of doctoral research related to the COVID-19 pandemic and, no doubt, planning for future pandemics.

Prioritisation of Patients and Safety Concerns

The safety of clinical trial participants is paramount for investigators and sponsors with regulatory agencies advocating flexibility within trial protocols during the pandemic [8]. Cancer patients are routinely classed as a vulnerable group due to the nature of the disease and treatment, but with the effects of SARS-CoV-2 infection unknown, all possible precautions were taken. A meta-analysis that assessed the effect of a cancer diagnosis on unvaccinated populations found a twofold increased risk of adverse outcomes (mortality, ICU admission and severity of COVID-19) in COVID-19 patients with cancer compared with those without cancer [9].

Reduced Recruitment

This concern for the safety of cancer patients meant that cancer patients were advised to isolate from the wider community to minimise the risk of contracting SARS-CoV-2 infection. Hospitals and healthcare facilities were one of the likeliest places to contract the infection due to the number of people admitted with SARS-CoV-2. Therefore, to reduce the risk, patients needed to avoid hospital. This caused difficulties for clinical trials, and the resultant missing data risked the quality of major trials. Some centres therefore led innovation to conduct more aspects remotely. Drugs were sent to patients' homes where they could be self-administered.

Remote consent and patient monitoring meant that patients who had previously been expected to travel long distances to trial centres on multiple occasions could now participate from the comfort and convenience of their own home [10]. The ability to innovate was experienced positively by research staff [10] and will hopefully mean that more patients will be able to participate in trials in the future as the time and cost to them are reduced. Now that these methods are available, it would be unethical to place additional burden on patients without good reason. These processes need to be flexible to account for inequalities in access to technology and digital literacy. There should be focus on freely given consent that accurately documents what the patient is consenting to [11].

Patients' concerns about safety were a potential barrier to recruitment during the pandemic where recruitment continued, but this was not always the case. One survey found that patients who chose to participate in clinical trials during the pandemic experienced increased anxiety, but their motivation (faith in their medical team, hope for a beneficial outcome or altruism) exceeded their anxiety [12]. A survey of gynaecological cancer patients found their fear of cancer progression to be worse than their fear of SARS-CoV-2 infection, and changes to their cancer care were a source of anxiety [13] which may have added to patients' motivation to continue to take part in clinical trials.

As clinical trials restarted, they were also affected by changes in treatment choices for standard of care. In early breast cancer, for example, a survey across 41 European countries showed an increase in surgery over systemic treatment for the primary systemic therapy in the first few months of the pandemic [14].

Changes to Treatment Regimens

Guidance provided by the European Society of Medical Oncology [15] provided a multidisciplinary consensus on the management of cancer patients during the pandemic. This was augmented by guidance for specific groups as well as national guidelines [16]. This included which patients should be prioritised for survival benefit and which treatment regimens required modifications (see Chap. 12 on SACT delivery). This guidance also had to be applied to clinical trials as appropriate by individual trial management groups. In the wait for guidance to emerge, many trials had paused, but restarting would prove difficult. Clinical research activity decreased suddenly in an effort to maintain patient safety [16]. Where a certain amount of risk would once have been deemed acceptable for patients taking part in clinical research, the additional risk of exposure to the SARS-CoV-2 virus with potentially fatal consequences was not. Investigators were faced with the difficult ethical decision as to whether the cancer or SARS-CoV-2 infection was a greater risk to individual patients. For early phase trials with a greater degree of uncertainty around the benefit to patients, this meant that many needed to be paused to recruitment. For patients already participating in clinical trials, there was an ethical duty to continue treatment as safely as possible. Guidance provided by the safety committees was discussed with patients on an individual basis to ensure continued informed consent.

The pandemic caused changes to some regimes to reduce patient visits and potential exposure to SARS-CoV-2. There was also the consideration of reduced capacity due to staff contracting the virus and treatment still needed to be delivered safely. For example, six-weekly dosing of pembrolizumab instead of three-weekly dosing was approved on the basis of preclinical data [17]. The clinical application of this new regimen in the real world then needed to be evaluated, creating further research opportunities. The new regimen demonstrated no difference in toxicity [18], so it has become standard practice with the benefit of increasing capacity in treatment units and reducing the travel and cost burden for patients. Hypofractionated radiation therapy was also applied when possible to limit hospital visits. This was done on a theoretical basis at times, requiring critical evaluation [19] providing further opportunities for cancer research.

Safety Monitoring

In addition to missing data due to patients not attending planned visits according to study protocols, central safety monitoring often undertaken by sponsors could no longer take place in person. The verification of source data had to be done remotely with no preparation and often without the required infrastructure [20]. This created the potential for increased data errors and reduced quality assurance [2]. Sponsor staff were also moved from other areas of research to focus on COVID-19 studies, so the number of staff available for the safety monitoring of cancer studies decreased. A lack of administrative staff due to sickness or isolation resulted in backlogs of typing reports and letters and delays in the filing of paper copies. Though the use of electronic systems was accelerated, there were inevitable delays in important safety information being recorded and reported.

Concurrent medications for the treatment of COVID will also have had an impact on safety monitoring owing to potential interactions or additional side effects. Toxicity reporting was also challenging as some effects of COVID-19 may not be easily distinguished from treatment toxicity, cancer symptoms or symptoms from other conditions. Identifying the cause of generic symptoms such as fatigue can be difficult at the best of times, and the absence of COVID-19 symptoms or a positive test (particularly in the first wave where testing was less reliable and there was limited availability) did not mean an absence of infection. When considering the vague presentation of some toxicities of immunotherapy, for example, these could be difficult to distinguish from the effects of COVID-19 or the vaccine. The variable and changing symptom profile of COVID-19 further contributed to this. The longer-term impacts of cancer treatments or late effects may also be confounded by the longer-term effects of COVID-19 causing difficulties in diagnosis.

Funding Cancer Research

In prioritising COVID-19 research, governments provided significant amounts of funding, but this came at a cost to other research. Money that would usually be available more generally for healthcare research was diverted to COVID-19. This forced many researchers to divert their research to consider COVID-19 or its impact on different aspects of society. The ongoing effect of the economic impact of the pandemic has meant that governments and major funding bodies including Horizon Europe and the European Research Council have planned significantly reduced budgets in subsequent years [21].

Charities that would usually fund healthcare research had to face the financial impact of public isolation measures. With businesses closed and public gatherings prohibited throughout Europe, raising money for charity became more difficult, and many charities also faced a further reduction of income as COVID-19 pandemic-related charities were set up, and the majority of public donations at the time went to those [2, 3, 22]. At the same time, many charities faced increased outgoings as existing commitments to charity staffing and outgoings, research infrastructure and ongoing projects had to be met. They then faced the increased costs associated with paused or delayed research. In the UK Cancer Research UK faced a fundraising shortfall of £120 m (€140 m) [3]. The UK charity lost approximately 25% of their overall income, and the Italian Foundation for Cancer Research (AIRC) and Spanish Association Against Cancer (AECC) experienced similar percentage losses [21]. The result of this income loss for cancer research is that many charities have made cuts to infrastructure and planned reduced budgets for subsequent years.

These reduced research budgets will reduce the amount of research that can take place. Important research questions that are not likely to be taken on by the pharmaceutical industry need these sources of funding. Research departments relying on these funding streams have made cuts, and there may unfortunately be a long-term effect on the workforce as more junior members of staff on less secure contracts have faced redundancy or sought employment elsewhere in the face of uncertainty.

Not all charities have faced such difficulties though. Some European cancer charities showed resilience by employing innovative virtual methods of fundraising, taking on staff with the skills to support this, including German Cancer Aid, the Norwegian Cancer Society and the Swedish Cancer Society [21]. The pandemic has highlighted the vital part that the charitable sector plays in cancer research, so to mitigate losses, governments, businesses and other corporations have assisted charities facing shortfalls.

Innovation in Cancer Research Resulting from the COVID-19 Pandemic

For all the negative effects of the pandemic, there was significant innovation within cancer research. Within research delivery, we have seen:

1. How barriers to research can be removed when required.
2. Research became mainstream, not just in healthcare but across society, and made headline news on a daily basis increasing societal awareness. Research participation is no longer unusual.
3. Accelerated innovation and use of digital methods to recruit and monitor patients including electronic consent.

4. The breadth of the skill set of cancer researchers and flexibility of the workforce to apply their knowledge and skills to other areas with little or no preparation.
5. Collaboration through virtual meetings; online data sharing has been accelerated, removing the need for costly face-to-face meetings and speeding up research processes.
6. Increased dissemination: conferences and meetings to share findings are now routinely held online or in hybrid format to reach a wider audience.

New opportunities to investigate altered treatment regimens have presented themselves which may lead to new standards of care. Regimens involving reduced patient visits have since been beneficial when rebuilding capacity to treat the increased number of patients presenting in the months and years after the main waves of the pandemic.

The scientific innovation related to research into the SARS-CoV-2 virus has also been repurposed to further cancer care. The technology used to develop the Oxford AstraZeneca SARS-CoV-2 vaccine is now being used to develop a vaccine-based treatment for lung cancer [23].

Conversely, understanding of the transmembrane serine protease 2 (TMPRSS2), a cell-surface protein that is expressed by epithelial cells of specific tissues including those in the aerodigestive tract that came from cancer research due to its relevance to prostate cancer was utilised in the understanding of the SARS-CoV-2 virus. [24]

Implications for Future Cancer Research

The resources put into SARS-CoV-2-related research demonstrate how quickly research can progress when funding is available, and there is prioritisation that lifts some of the barriers that come with research governance. The successes are the treatments and vaccinations for the virus that have saved countless lives. The publicity around SARS-CoV-2 research reached every household. Research in general is no longer something that a small number of patients come into contact with, and hopefully, this has embedded research into routine practice, where more patients are offered, ask about and take up the opportunity to take part in clinical research.

Following the pandemic, when designing research, risk mitigation related to pandemic situations is routinely considered, and the ongoing effects of the COVID-19 pandemic in the population may need to be considered. The legacy of patients being diagnosed with cancer later due to isolation measures and lack of resources will also affect the population coming forward for cancer trials in the coming years. There may be a greater number of patients with advanced disease suitable for trials than those with early cancers.

Safety concerns related to vaccines and treatments for SARS-CoV-2 were raised on social media outlets due to the speed at which the research took place, but the large number of exposed individuals made the recruitment of a large number of patients very easy. Unfortunately large cancer trials to test one or two drugs are harder to accomplish as genomics show us that cancer is a collection of diseases. Cancer research will therefore be limited by the heterogeneity of the disease, but lessons learned in the delivery of research can increase the rate of delivery and innovation.

References

1. Poggio F, Tagliamento M, Di Maio M, Martelli V, De Maria A, Barisione E, Grosso M, Boccardo F, Pronzato P, Del Mastro L, Lambertini M (2020) Assessing the Impact of the COVID-19 Outbreak on the Attitudes and Practice of Italian Oncologists Toward Breast Cancer Care and Related Research Activities. JCO Oncol Pract 16(11):e1304–e1314. https://doi.org/10.1200/OP.20.00297
2. Auletta JJ, Adamson PC, Agin JE, Kearns P, Kennedy S, Kieran MW, Ludwinski DM, Knox LJ, McKay K, Rhiner P, Thiele CJ, Cripe TP (2020) Pediatric cancer research: Surviving COVID-19. Pediatr Blood Cancer 67(9):e28435. https://doi.org/10.1002/pbc.28435
3. Cancer Research UK (2020) The fundraising and organisational challenges faced by the charitable and voluntary sector during the COVID-19 pandemic—a Cancer Research UK briefing. Available from: https://www.cancerresearchuk.org/sites/default/files/cancer_research_uk_-_april_charity_fundraising_briefing_england.pdf. Accessed 25th June 2023
4. Penel N, Hammoudi A, Marliot G, De Courreges A, Cucchi M, Mirabel X, Leblanc E, Lartigau E (2021) Major impact of COVID-19 national containment on activities in the French northern comprehensive cancer center. Med Oncol 38(3):28. https://doi.org/10.1007/s12032-021-01467-0
5. Lancet T (2021) Genomic sequencing in pandemics. Lancet 397(10273):445. https://doi.org/10.1016/S0140-6736(21)00257-9
6. Park JJH, Mogg R, Smith GE, Nakimuli-Mpungu E, Jehan F, Rayner CR, Condo J, Decloedt EH, Nachega JB, Reis G, Mills EJ (2021) How COVID-19 has fundamentally changed clinical research in global health. Lancet Glob Health 9(5):e711–e720. https://doi.org/10.1016/S2214-109X(20)30542-8
7. Bailey C, Black JRM, Swanton C (2020) Cancer research: the lessons to learn from COVID-19. Cancer Discov 10(9):1263–1266. https://doi.org/10.1158/2159-8290.CD-20-0823
8. Saini KS, de Las HB, de Castro J, Venkitaraman R, Poelman M, Srinivasan G, Saini ML, Verma S, Leone M, Aftimos P, Curigliano G (2020) Effect of the COVID-19 pandemic on cancer treatment and research. Lancet Haematol 7(6):e432–e435. https://doi.org/10.1016/S2352-3026(20)30123-X
9. Di Felice G, Visci G, Teglia F, Angelini M, Boffetta P (2022) Effect of cancer on outcome of COVID-19 patients: a systematic review and meta-analysis of studies of unvaccinated patients. elife 11:e74634. https://doi.org/10.7554/eLife.74634
10. Hood B, Boyd R, Crowe T, Turner K, Wellman S, Brown H, Johnson A (2022) Effect of COVID-19 on cancer research nursing services. Cancer Nursing Pract 22:e1821. https://doi.org/10.7748/cnp.2022.e1821
11. Doherty GJ, Goksu M, de Paula BHR (2020) Rethinking cancer clinical trials for COVID-19 and beyond. Nat Cancer 1(6):568–572. https://doi.org/10.1038/s43018-020-0083-x
12. Hood B (2023) Understanding the experiences of cancer patients referred for a clinical trial during the COVID-19 pandemic. British J Nursing 32(2):2052–2819. Available from: https://www.britishjournalofnursing.com/content/professional/understanding-the-experiences-of-cancer-patients-referred-for-a-clinical-trial-during-the-covid-19-pandemic. Accessed 25th June 2023
13. Gultekin M, Ak S, Ayhan A, Strojna A, Pletnev A, Fagotti A, Perrone AM, Erzeneoglu BE, Temiz BE, Lemley B, Soyak B, Hughes C, Cibula D, Haidopoulos D, Brennan D, Cola E, van der Steen-Banasik E, Urkmez E, Akilli H, Zapardiel I, Tóth I, Sehouli J, Zalewski K, Bahremand

K, Chiva L, Mirza MR, Papageorgiou M, Zoltan N, Adámková P, Morice P, Garrido-Mallach S, Akgor U, Theodoulidis V, Arik Z, Steffensen KD, Fotopoulou C (2021) Perspectives, fears and expectations of patients with gynaecological cancers during the COVID-19 pandemic: a Pan-European study of the European Network of Gynaecological Cancer Advocacy Groups (ENGAGe). Cancer Med 10(1):208–219. https://doi.org/10.1002/cam4.3605
14. Gasparri ML, Gentilini OD, Lueftner D, Kuehn T, Kaidar-Person O, Poortmans P (2020) Changes in breast cancer management during the Corona Virus Disease 19 pandemic: an international survey of the European Breast Cancer Research Association of Surgical Trialists (EUBREAST). Breast 52:110–115. https://doi.org/10.1016/j.breast.2020.05.006
15. Curigliano G, Banerjee S, Cervantes A, Garassino MC, Garrido P, Girard N, Haanen J, Jordan K, Lordick F, Machiels JP, Michielin O, Peters S, Tabernero J, Douillard JY, Pentheroudakis G, Panel members (2020) Managing cancer patients during the COVID-19 pandemic: an ESMO multidisciplinary expert consensus. Ann Oncol 31(10):1320–1335. https://doi.org/10.1016/j.annonc.2020.07.010
16. Petrova D, Pérez-Gómez B, Pollán M, Sánchez MJ (2020) Implications of the COVID-19 pandemic for cancer in Spain. Med Clin (Engl Ed) 155(6):263–266. https://doi.org/10.1016/j.medcle.2020.04.018
17. Lala M, Li TR, de Alwis DP, Sinha V, Mayawala K, Yamamoto N, Siu LL, Chartash E, Aboshady H, Jain L (2020) A six-weekly dosing schedule for pembrolizumab in patients with cancer based on evaluation using modelling and simulation. Eur J Cancer 131:68–75. https://doi.org/10.1016/j.ejca.2020.02.016
18. Douglas C, Lord H (2021) P34.01 6-weekly vs 3-weekly Pembrolizumab—toxicities and tolerance in the COVID-era. J Thorac Oncol 16(10):S1059–S1060. https://doi.org/10.1016/j.jtho.2021.08.418
19. Portaluri M, Barba MC, Musio D, Tramacere F, Pati F, Bambace S (2020) Hypofractionation in COVID-19 radiotherapy: a mix of evidence based medicine and of opportunities. Radiother Oncol 150:191–194. https://doi.org/10.1016/j.radonc.2020.06.036
20. Rubio-San-Simón A, André N, Cefalo MG, Aerts I, Castañeda A, Benezech S, Makin G, van Eijkelenburg N, Nysom K, Marshall L, Gambart M, Hladun R, Rossig C, Bergamaschi L, Fagioli F, Carpenter B, Ducassou S, Owens C, Øra I, Ribelles AJ, De Wilde B, Guerra-García P, Strullu M, Rizzari C, Ek T, Hettmer S, Gerber NU, Rawlings C, Diezi M, Palmu S, Ruggiero A, Verdú J, de Rojas T, Vassal G, Geoerger B, Moreno L, Bautista F (2020) Impact of COVID-19 in paediatric early-phase cancer clinical trials in Europe: a report from the Innovative Therapies for Children with Cancer (ITCC) consortium. Eur J Cancer 141:82–91. https://doi.org/10.1016/j.ejca.2020.09.024
21. Tsagakis I, Papatriantafyllou M (2020) Safeguarding cancer research funding by European charities amidst the COVID-19 pandemic. Mol Oncol 14(12):2987–2993. https://doi.org/10.1002/1878-0261.12839
22. Cancer Research UK (2022) Annual report and accounts 2021/22. Available from: https://www.cancerresearchuk.org/sites/default/files/annualreports21-22.pdf. Accessed 25th Jun 2023
23. McAuliffe J, Chan HF, Noblecourt L, Ramirez-Valdez RA, Pereira-Almeida V, Zhou Y, Pollock E, Cappuccini F, Redchenko I, Hill AV, Leung CSK, Van den Eynde BJ (2021) Heterologous prime-boost vaccination targeting MAGE-type antigens promotes tumor T-cell infiltration and improves checkpoint blockade therapy. J Immunother Cancer 9(9):e003218. https://doi.org/10.1136/jitc-2021-003218
24. Stopsack KH, Mucci LA, Antonarakis ES, Nelson PS, Kantoff PW (2020) TMPRSS2 and COVID-19: Serendipity or Opportunity for Intervention? Cancer Discov 10(6):779–782. https://doi.org/10.1158/2159-8290.CD-20-0451

Recommended Reading

Bakouny Z, Labaki C, Bhalla S, Schmidt AL, Steinharter JA, Cocco J, Tremblay DA, Awad MM, Kessler A, Haddad RI, Evans M, Busser F, Wotman M, Curran CR, Zimmerman BS, Bouchard G, Jun T, Nuzzo PV, Qin Q, Hirsch L, Feld J, Kelleher KM, Seidman D, Huang H, Anderson-Keightly HM, El Zarif T, Alaiwi SA, Champagne C, Rosenbloom TD, Stewart PS, Johnson BE, Trinh Q, Tolaney SM, Galsky MD, Choueiri TK, Doroshow DB (2022) Oncology clinical trial disruption during the COVID-19 pandemic: a COVID-19 and cancer outcomes study. Ann Oncol 33(8):836–844. https://doi.org/10.1016/j.annonc.2022.04.071. Epub 2022 Jun 14. PMID: 35715285; PMCID: PMC9197329

Desai A, Gainor JF, Hegde A, Schram AM, Curigliano G, Pal S, Liu SV, Halmos B, Groisberg R, Grande E, Dragovich T, Matrana M, Agarwal N, Chawla S, Kato S, Morgan G, Kasi PM, Solomon B, Loong HH, Park H, Choueiri TK, Subbiah IM, Pemmaraju N, Subbiah V (2021) COVID19 and Cancer Clinical Trials Working Group. COVID-19 vaccine guidance for patients with cancer participating in oncology clinical trials. Nat Rev Clin Oncol 18(5):313–319. https://doi.org/10.1038/s41571-021-00487-z. Epub 2021 Mar 15. Erratum in: Nat Rev Clin Oncol. 2021 Mar 23;: PMID: 33723371; PMCID: PMC7957448

Hood B, Boyd R, Crowe T, Turner K, Wellman S, Brown H, Johnson A (2022) Effect of COVID-19 on cancer research nursing services. Cancer Nursing Pract 22:e1821. https://doi.org/10.7748/cnp.2022.e1821

Postel-Vinay S, Massard C, Soria JC (2020) Coronavirus disease (COVID-19) outbreak and phase 1 trials: should we consider a specific patient management? Eur J Cancer 137:235–239. https://doi.org/10.1016/j.ejca.2020.07.009. Epub 2020 Jul 27. PMID: 32805640; PMCID: PMC7383132

Shiely F, Foley J, Stone A, Cobbe E, Browne S, Murphy E, Kelsey M, Walsh-Crowley J, Eustace JA (2021) Managing clinical trials during COVID-19: experience from a clinical research facility. Trials 22(1):62. https://doi.org/10.1186/s13063-020-05004-8

Tagliamento M, Poggio F, Perachino M, Pirrone C, Fregatti P, Lambertini M (2022) The evolving scenario of cancer care provision across the COVID-19 pandemic in Europe. Curr Opin Support Palliat Care 16(3):110–116. https://doi.org/10.1097/SPC.0000000000000601

Zimmerman S (2020) Challenges in managing clinical trials in oncology in the COVID-19 Era. Available from: https://www.esmo.org/oncology-news/challenges-in-managing-clinical-trials-in-oncology-in-the-covid-19-era. Accessed 25 June 2023

Open Access This chapter is licensed under the terms of the Creative Commons Attribution 4.0 International License (http://creativecommons.org/licenses/by/4.0/), which permits use, sharing, adaptation, distribution and reproduction in any medium or format, as long as you give appropriate credit to the original author(s) and the source, provide a link to the Creative Commons license and indicate if changes were made.

The images or other third party material in this chapter are included in the chapter's Creative Commons license, unless indicated otherwise in a credit line to the material. If material is not included in the chapter's Creative Commons license and your intended use is not permitted by statutory regulation or exceeds the permitted use, you will need to obtain permission directly from the copyright holder.

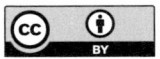

Haematological Perspectives on COVID-19 and Cancer

3

Karen Sayal

Check Your Knowledge and Experience
1. What are the most common direct haematological complications of cancer?
2. What changes have been made to neutropenic sepsis protocol in your local healthcare setting?
3. What strategies can be employed to help guide and support cancer patients as they navigate the dual challenge of cancer treatment during a pandemic?

Introduction

The COVID-19 pandemic has had an immense impact on healthcare systems with unique challenges presented for cancer patients. This chapter aims to explore the direct haematological implications of SARS-CoV-2 infection in cancer patients as well as the indirect effects on patient management, such as changes in treatment protocols and the management of neutropenic sepsis. We present an overview of the key haematological considerations in the complex relationship between SARS-CoV-2 and cancer.

Direct Haematological Effects of COVID-19 in Cancer Patients

Increased Risk of Thromboembolic Events

Pathophysiology
SARS-CoV-2 has been shown to be associated with an increased risk of thromboembolic events in cancer patients [1]. The underlying pathophysiology involves a complex interplay between the SARS-CoV-2 virus, systemic inflammation and

---

K. Sayal (✉)
Department of Oncology, University College London Hospitals NHS Foundation Trust, London, UK

coagulation abnormalities. SARS-CoV-2 primarily targets endothelial cells by binding to angiotensin-converting enzyme 2 (ACE2) [2], leading to endothelial dysfunction and microvascular injury. This in turn promotes a pro-inflammatory and pro-thrombotic state characterised by the activation of the coagulation cascade, platelet aggregation and fibrin deposition.

Furthermore, the immune response to SARS-CoV-2 infection can lead to a cytokine storm characterised by the release of large amounts of pro-inflammatory cytokines, such as interleukin-6 (IL-6), tumour necrosis factor-alpha (TNF-α) and interleukin-1 beta (IL-1β) [3]. This heightened inflammatory state can cause an imbalance in coagulation factors and anticoagulant mechanisms, resulting in a hypercoagulable state.

Cancer patients are already at an increased risk of developing thromboembolic events due to cancer-specific factors, such as the release of procoagulant factors by tumour cells, treatment-induced endothelial damage and immobilisation. The additional risk posed by SARS-CoV-2 infection further exacerbates the thrombotic risk in this population.

Clinical Manifestations

The clinical manifestations of thromboembolic events in cancer patients with SARS-CoV-2 can range from asymptomatic cases to life-threatening complications. The most common thrombotic events include deep vein thrombosis (DVT), pulmonary embolism (PE) and arterial thrombosis.

DVT typically presents with unilateral leg pain, swelling and erythema. PE may manifest as a sudden onset of shortness of breath, chest pain or tachycardia. However, it is important to note that these classical signs can overlap with symptoms directly associated with the underlying malignancy, thereby making diagnosis more challenging. Arterial thrombosis can lead to acute limb ischaemia, cerebrovascular events or myocardial infarctions depending upon the affected arterial bed.

Management and Prevention Strategies

The management of thromboembolic events in cancer patients with SARS-CoV-2 infection involves a multidisciplinary approach which includes risk stratification, anticoagulation therapy and close monitoring. The guiding principles for diagnosis and management of suspected DVT are summarised in Fig. 3.1 [4].

For patients at high risk of thromboembolism, prophylactic anticoagulation with low molecular weight heparin (LMWH) or direct oral anticoagulants (DOACs) may be considered.

For patients who develop a thromboembolic event, therapeutic anticoagulation with LMWH, unfractionated heparin or DOACs are the mainstay of treatment; in certain more complex cases, additional interventions such as catheter-directed thrombolysis, mechanical thrombectomy or an inferior vena cava (IVC) filter placement may be required.

Preventative measures include early mobilisation, adequate hydration and patient education on the signs and symptoms of thromboembolic events. Additionally, the clinical team should carefully evaluate the risk-benefit profile of cancer therapeutics

Venous thromboembolism: diagnosis and anticoagulation treatment

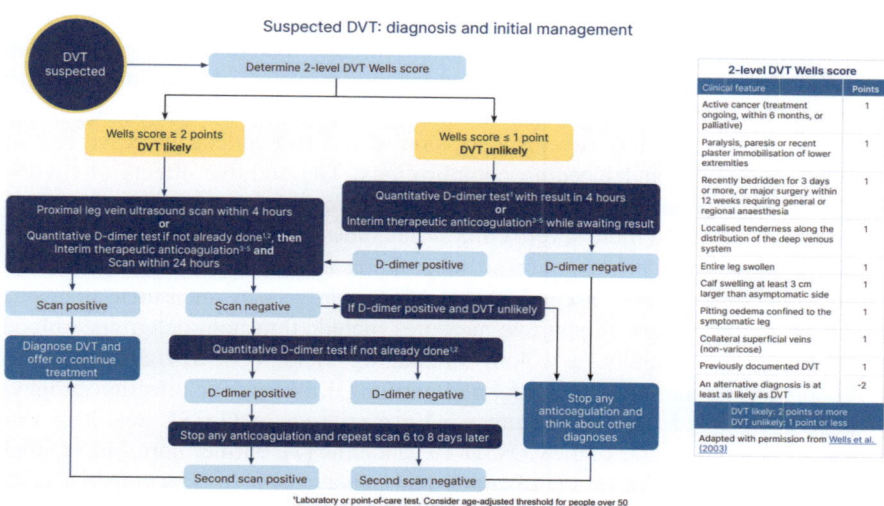

Fig. 3.1 The clinical workflow for the diagnosis and management of suspected DVT (Reproduced courtesy of the National Institute for Health and Care Excellence)

and consider dose adjustments or alternative treatment options to minimise thrombotic risk if appropriate.

Bone Marrow Suppression and Pancytopenia

COVID-19-Related Cytokine Storm

One of the most significant complications of SARS-CoV-2 infection is the development of a cytokine storm [5]. A cytokine storm is characterised by the uncontrolled release of pro-inflammatory cytokines such as IL-6, IL-8, vascular endothelial growth factor (VEGF) and monocyte chemoattractant protein-1 (MCP-1). The overwhelming immune response can lead to widespread tissue damage and organ dysfunction which includes haematopoietic systemic involvement with subsequent bone marrow suppression.

Bone marrow suppression due to a cytokine storm can result in pancytopenia, a condition characterised by a decrease of all three major blood cell lineages: red blood cells, white blood cells and platelets. The exact mechanisms by which SARS-CoV-2-related cytokine storm induces bone marrow suppression still remains unclear [6]. However, it is postulated that high levels of pro-inflammatory cytokines may directly inhibit haematopoietic progenitor cell proliferation and differentiation. Alternatively, indirect bone marrow damage may be induced through the release of reactive oxygen species.

Implications for Cancer Patients

Cancer patients are particularly vulnerable to the wider implications of bone marrow suppression due to a combination of the primary malignancy in combination with the myelosuppressive effect of cytotoxic treatments which form the mainstay of oncological care. Chemotherapy, radiation therapy and a subset of targeted therapeutics can directly cause myelosuppression with a subsequent increased risk of infections, anaemia and bleeding complications. The additive effects of SARS-CoV-2-related cytokine storm on bone marrow suppression can further exacerbate these risks and lead to more severe clinical outcomes in cancer patients.

The management of bone marrow suppression in cancer patients with SARS-CoV-2 infection requires a combination of supportive care measures alongside treatment modifications. Supportive measures include threshold-determined blood transfusions and granulocyte colony-stimulating factor (G-CSF) administration with appropriate antibiotic, antiviral and antifungal therapy for infection prophylaxis/treatment. Indeed, the recommended use criteria for G-CSF treatment was expanded over the course of the COVID-19 pandemic [7]. Furthermore, closer monitoring to ensure the early identification and management of pancytopenia is an important component in optimising clinical outcomes and reducing morbidity and mortality.

The Direct Link Between COVID-19 and Malignancies

The interplay between SARS-CoV-2 infection and malignancies is complex. In the next section, we will focus on the discussion of the key factors underpinning such dynamics. Breast cancer as a representative example of a solid malignancy and haematological malignancies will be explored.

Impact of COVID-19 on Cancer Progression

COVID-19 infection may have direct effects on breast cancer progression through various mechanisms. SARS-CoV-2 utilises the angiotensin-converting enzyme 2 (ACE2) receptor to enter epithelial cells. ACE2 is widely expressed in various tissues, including breast tissue and certain breast cancer subtypes. It has been suggested that the interaction between SARS-CoV-2 and ACE2 may contribute to breast cancer progression by modulating the local renin-angiotensin system (RAS) which plays a role in tumour growth, angiogenesis and metastasis [8].

It has been suggested that breast cancer patients with higher ACE2 expression levels may be more susceptible to SARS-CoV-2 infection which may then potentially affect cancer progression [9]. Furthermore, the ACE2 receptor has been found to be upregulated in specific breast cancer subtypes, such as triple-negative breast cancer (TNBC), suggesting a potential association between SARS-CoV-2 infection and more aggressive breast cancer subtypes [9].

The systemic inflammatory response triggered by SARS-CoV-2 may alter the growth trajectory of tumours by simulating angiogenesis, matrix remodelling and expression of adhesion factors [10]. All of these processes can contribute to tumour cell invasion and dissemination. In addition, the dysregulated immune response to SARS-CoV-2 could potentially impair the immune system's ability to recognise and eliminate tumour cells, thereby facilitating tumour progression. Further investigation is required to shed light on these potentially pathogenic drivers and evaluate their role and impact on patient prognosis and overall clinical outcomes.

Impact of COVID-19 Specific to Haematological Malignancies

Haematological malignancies, such as leukaemia, lymphoma and myeloma, originate in the bone marrow or lymphatic systems. Haematological malignancies typically affect the immune system in a more profound manner than solid tumours.

As a consequence, patients with haematological malignancies are more likely to present with more severe haematological abnormalities of SARS-CoV-2 infection compared to solid tumours [11]. Patients may experience prolonged neutropenia or severe lymphopenia, conditions characterised by low levels of neutrophils or lymphocytes, respectively [11]. Patients may also experience increased anaemia or thrombocytopenia due to generalised dysfunction of the bone marrow [11].

SARS-CoV-2 mortality in patients with haematological malignancies has been shown to be higher than in the solid tumour setting [12]. The higher mortality is due to the severe compromise on the immune system which arises in a disease-direct manner [12]. Innate and adaptive immune responses are attenuated, resulting in an increased risk of severe infective complications such as pneumonia, acute respiratory distress syndrome (ARDS) or multi-organ failure. In addition, patients with haematological malignancies undergo profoundly immunosuppressive treatments, such as stem cell transplantation, which further compounds the widespread immunosuppressive impact of the malignancy.

Indirect Haematological Effects of SARS-CoV-2 in Cancer Patients

In this section, we will discuss the indirect haematological implications of SARS-CoV-2 infection on cancer management. We will focus on neutropenic sepsis, a common complication of cancer treatment, pandemic-related delays in treatment delivery and the effect of the pandemic on the mental well-being of cancer patients.

Neutropenic Sepsis

The COVID-19 pandemic led to significant changes in the management of neutropenic sepsis in cancer patients. Healthcare systems had to adapt to the challenges posed by the pandemic, including new infection control measures with additional strains on the use of healthcare resources which had implications on the neutropenic sepsis workflow.

Neutropenic sepsis is a potentially life-threatening complication of cancer treatment. It occurs when an immunosuppressed patient develops a systemic infection

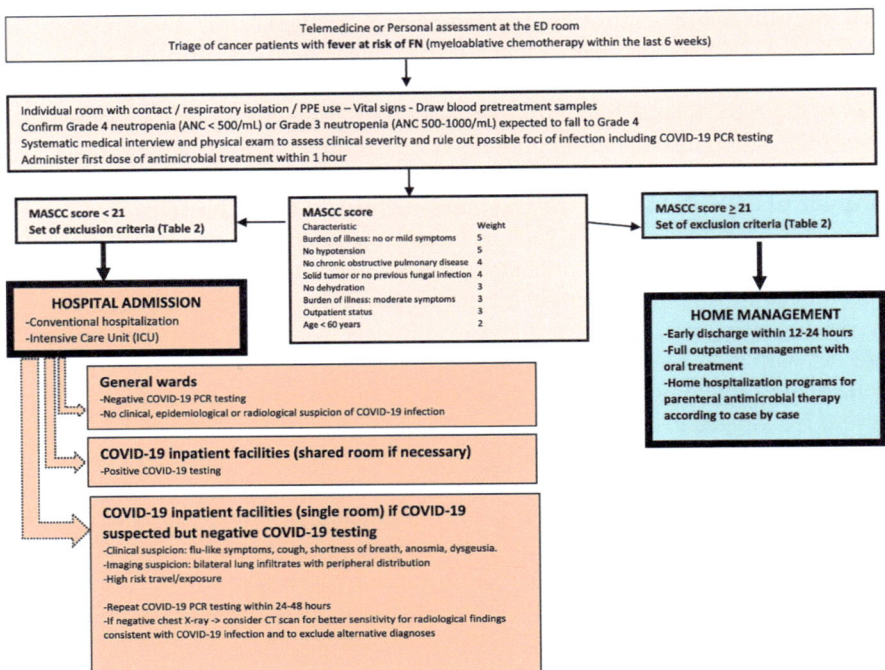

Fig. 3.2 The diagnosis and preliminary management of patients with suspected neutropenic sepsis over the course of the COVID-19 pandemic (Reproduced with permission from Springer Nature ~~courtesy of~~ Cooksley et al)

due to neutropenia. Neutropenic sepsis and SARS-CoV-2 infection have overlapping clinical features. Common presenting symptoms include fever, respiratory symptoms, cough and signs of systemic inflammation. It can therefore be difficult to have diagnostic certainty in such circumstances which may then potentially delay the most appropriate treatment route. A representative example of the typical clinical workflow is shown in Fig. 3.2 [13].

In response to the pandemic, healthcare systems made adjustments to the neutropenic sepsis management guidelines. Such changes included:

(a) Telemedicine: The increased use of telemedicine allowed clinical teams to monitor patients remotely, thereby helping to identify neutropenic sepsis at an earlier stage, instigate earlier treatment and provide tailored remote clinical guidance to patients.
(b) Outpatient management: Due to the risk of hospital-acquired COVID-19 infection, there was an increased focus on the outpatient management of neutropenic sepsis in selected low-risk patients [14]. Outpatient treatment involved oral antibiotics, increased self-monitoring and guidance on seeking immediate input in the event of a clinical deterioration.

(c) Inpatient management: Care involved a balance between the need for rapid treatment of neutropenic sepsis whilst minimising the risk of COVID-19 exposure for patients. A range of enhanced infection control measures, such as isolation protocols and the use of personal protective equipment (PPE), were implemented. Dedicated wards were also established for COVID-19 confirmed-positive patients in order to separate infected and uninfected patients, thereby offering further protection for vulnerable cancer patients. Visitor policies were restricted to limit transmission potential which included visitor number restrictions, screening visitors for symptoms and requiring visitors to wear masks and follow hand hygiene protocols.

Delays in Diagnosis and Treatment Due to the COVID-19 Pandemic

An indirect effect of the COVID-19 pandemic on cancer patients has been the consequential delay in diagnosis and treatment. The pandemic has led to widespread disruption in oncological services, including the postponement of routine cancer screening programmes and limited access to diagnostic imaging and biopsies [15]. Such delays may also result in disease presenting at more advanced stages of progression such as bone marrow infiltration, thereby leading to poorer clinical outcomes [15].

Adjustments to cancer treatment protocols were required over the course of the pandemic in order to minimise patients' risk of SARS-CoV-2 exposure and complications. Such amendments included operative delays, prioritisation of neoadjuvant therapies and a preference towards less myelosuppressive systemic regimens. The longer-term implications for tumour control and survival outcomes remain to be determined.

Mental Health Implications and Quality of Lifestyle

The pandemic had a significant impact on the mental health and quality of life of cancer patients. The associated chronic stress has consequential impacts on global immune and haematological function as well as adherence to intense myelosuppressive treatment protocols.

Cancer patients experienced increased anxiety and depression during the pandemic [16]. The fear of contracting SARS-CoV-2 and the uncertainty surrounding treatment plans led to increased feelings of anxiety and depression amongst patients which could exacerbate existing mental health conditions or trigger new conditions.

The need for social distancing measures and the potential for prolonged periods of isolation further contributed to feelings of loneliness amongst patients [17]. In such circumstances, support from family, friends, support groups, counselling and rehabilitation programmes was significantly curtailed, resulting in a more profound effect on the patient's mental well-being.

Conclusion

In conclusion, the COVID-19 pandemic has had significant direct and indirect haematological implications for cancer patients. Direct effects include an increased risk of thromboembolic events and coagulation abnormalities as well as bone marrow suppression and pancytopenia resulting from COVID-19-related cytokine storm. Furthermore, SARS-CoV-2 may have a direct impact on cancer progression as exemplified by its potential influence on breast cancer subtypes.

Indirect effects of the pandemic involved changes in the management of neutropenic sepsis, changes in diagnostic and treatment pathways and the psychological implications for cancer patients. Healthcare systems have adapted to the pandemic by utilising telemedicine, harnessing strategies for optimising outpatient management and increasing inpatient infection control measures. General disruption to oncological services has impacted the diagnostic and treatment pathways which has had an impact on the overall patient experience.

The complex relationship between SARS-CoV-2 infection and cancer highlighted the need for the continued development of innovative approaches to optimise patient care as we transitioned into the post-pandemic era of cancer care.

Test Your Learning
1. What are the three main haematological complications associated with SARS-CoV-2 in cancer patients?
2. How has the COVID-19 pandemic affected cancer treatment schedules and patient outcomes?
3. What role does mental health play in the overall well-being of cancer patients during the pandemic, and how can healthcare professional best support patients?

References

1. Alpert N, Rapp JL, Marcellino B, Lieberman-Cribbin W, Flores R, Taioli E (2021) Clinical course of cancer patients with COVID-19: a retrospective cohort study. JNCI Cancer Spectrum 5(1):pkaa085. https://doi.org/10.1093/jncics/pkaa085
2. Wrapp D, Wang N, Corbett KS, Goldsmith JA, Hsieh C-L, Abiona O, Graham BS, McLellan JS (2020) Cryo-EM structure of the 2019-NCoV spike in the Prefusion conformation. Science (New York, NY) 367(6483):1260–1263. https://doi.org/10.1126/science.abb2507
3. Schurink B, Roos E, Radonic T, Barbe E, Bouman CSC, de Boer HH, de Bree GJ et al (2020) Viral presence and immunopathology in patients with lethal COVID-19: a prospective autopsy cohort study. Lancet Microbe 1(7):e290–e299. https://doi.org/10.1016/S2666-5247(20)30144-0
4. National Institute for Health and Care Excellence (2020) Venous thromboembolic diseases: diagnosis, management and thrombophilia testing. https://www.nice.org.uk/guidance/ng158/resources/visual-summary-pdf-11193380893
5. Hong R, Zhao H, Yiyun Wang Y, Chen HC, Yongxian H, Wei G, Huang H (2021) Clinical characterization and risk factors associated with cytokine release syndrome induced by COVID-19 and chimeric antigen receptor T-cell therapy. Bone Marrow Transplant 56(3):570–580. https://doi.org/10.1038/s41409-020-01060-5

6. Wang X, Wen Y, Xie X, Liu Y, Tan X, Cai Q, Zhang Y et al (2021) Dysregulated hematopoiesis in bone marrow Marks severe COVID-19. Cell Discover 7(1):1–18. https://doi.org/10.1038/s41421-021-00296-9
7. Curigliano G, Banerjee S, Cervantes A, Garassino MC, Garrido P, Girard N, Haanen J et al (2020) Managing cancer patients during the COVID-19 pandemic: an ESMO multidisciplinary expert consensus. Ann Oncol 31(10):1320–1335. https://doi.org/10.1016/j.annonc.2020.07.010
8. Francescangeli F, De Angelis ML, Zeuner A (2020) COVID-19: a potential driver of immune-mediated breast cancer recurrence? Breast Cancer Res 22(1):117. https://doi.org/10.1186/s13058-020-01360-0
9. Nair MG, Prabhu JS, Sridhar TS (2021) High expression of ACE2 in HER2 subtype of breast cancer is a marker of poor prognosis. Cancer Treat Res Commun 27:100321. https://doi.org/10.1016/j.ctarc.2021.100321
10. Caccuri F, Bugatti A, Zani A, De Palma A, Di Silvestre D, Manocha E, Filippini F et al (2021) SARS-CoV-2 infection remodels the phenotype and promotes angiogenesis of primary human lung endothelial cells. Microorganisms 9(7):1438. https://doi.org/10.3390/microorganisms9071438
11. Langerbeins P, Hallek M (2022) COVID-19 in patients with hematologic malignancy. Blood 140(3):236–252. https://doi.org/10.1182/blood.2021012251
12. Hardy N, Vegivinti CTR, Mehta M, Thurnham J, Mebane A, Pederson JM, Tarchand R et al (2023) Mortality of COVID-19 in patients with hematological malignancies versus solid tumors: a systematic literature review and meta-analysis. Clin Exp Med 23:1–15. https://doi.org/10.1007/s10238-023-01004-5
13. Cooksley T, Font C, Scotte F, Escalante C, Johnson L, Anderson R, Rapoport B (2021) Emerging challenges in the evaluation of fever in cancer patients at risk of febrile neutropenia in the era of COVID-19: a MASCC position paper. Support Care Cancer 29(2):1129–1138. https://doi.org/10.1007/s00520-020-05906-y
14. Baus CJ, Kelley B, Dow-Hillgartner E, Kyriakopoulos CE, Schulz LT, Lepak AJ, LoConte NK (2023) Neutropenic fever–associated admissions among patients with solid tumors receiving chemotherapy during the COVID-19 pandemic. JAMA Netw Open 6(3):e234881. https://doi.org/10.1001/jamanetworkopen.2023.4881
15. İlgün AS, Özmen V (2021) The impact of the COVID-19 pandemic on breast cancer patients. European J Breast Health 18(1):85–90. https://doi.org/10.4274/ejbh.galenos.2021.2021-11-5
16. Tolia M, Symvoulakis EK, Matalliotakis E, Kamekis A, Adamou M, Kountourakis P, Mauri D et al (2023) COVID-19 emotional and mental impact on cancer patients receiving radiotherapy: an interpretation of potential explaining descriptors. Curr Oncol 30(1):586–597. https://doi.org/10.3390/curroncol30010046
17. González-Sanguino C, Ausín B, Castellanos MÁ, Saiz J, López-Gómez A, Ugidos C, Muñoz M (2020) Mental health consequences during the initial stage of the 2020 coronavirus pandemic (COVID-19) in Spain. Brain Behav Immun 87:172–176. https://doi.org/10.1016/j.bbi.2020.05.040

Open Access This chapter is licensed under the terms of the Creative Commons Attribution 4.0 International License (http://creativecommons.org/licenses/by/4.0/), which permits use, sharing, adaptation, distribution and reproduction in any medium or format, as long as you give appropriate credit to the original author(s) and the source, provide a link to the Creative Commons license and indicate if changes were made.

The images or other third party material in this chapter are included in the chapter's Creative Commons license, unless indicated otherwise in a credit line to the material. If material is not included in the chapter's Creative Commons license and your intended use is not permitted by statutory regulation or exceeds the permitted use, you will need to obtain permission directly from the copyright holder.

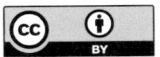

Telehealth, Digital Technology and the COVID-19 Pandemic, the Impact on Cancer Care

Mark Foulkes

Check Your Experience

If you work in healthcare, how has the increased use of technology changed your working day over the course of the COVID-19 pandemic?

What types of technology have been employed during the pandemic to continue to deliver cancer care?

Introduction

As the novel coronavirus pandemic took hold in 2020, with the need to socially isolate, there was a greater shift to the use of technology in order to continue to perform everyday tasks. Education, shopping socialising and employment all began to be carried out using digital solutions.

Healthcare embraced similar solutions in order to maintain oversight, and the delivery of patient care and cancer care was certainly not insulated from this [1]. Fairly soon after the pandemic began, most countries with well-developed health systems began to try and balance the need to continue to treat cancers, sometimes urgently, against the requirement to minimise exposure of patients and hospital staff to SARS-CoV-2 infection, whilst also balancing potential increased effects in the cancer population of infection with the virus.

Five years after the emergence of the SARS-CoV-2 virus, it would be useful to appraise the widespread use of digital technology in cancer care, the effectiveness of this and the overall effect on patient experience.

M. Foulkes (✉)
Macmillan Lead Cancer Nurse and Nurse Consultant,
Royal Berkshire NHS Foundation Trust, Reading, UK
e-mail: mark.foulkes@royalberkshire.nhs.uk

Collaboration and Data Sharing Using Digital Platforms and the Use of 'Big Data'

Soon after the first wave of the pandemic began to sweep around the world in March 2020, the benefits of sharing information about the virus and how it affected discrete populations of patients became obvious. It was also clear that the technology needed to collect and store huge quantities of data was already in place and could be accessed via academic institutions and other organisations. It therefore became possible for individuals to enter 'live-time' data about symptoms, treatments and responses to these treatments.

One of the best-known and most widely used database studies of this type outside of cancer is the Zoe Covid Symptom Study [2]. This was is a symptom reporting app employed in epidemiological research whereby members of the general public reported their health status each day with a focus on identifying those individuals who are displaying symptoms of COVID-19. Within one day of being launched in the United Kingdom in March 2020, the app had been downloaded more than a million times. The Covid Symptom Study continued to collect more than a million sets of individual data per day throughout 2020 and 2021 and continued to do so until 2022. The study's huge database allowed the researchers to first identify the loss of taste or smell as an important symptom of COVID-19 as well as to identify vaccinated individuals who had less severe infections than those who remained unvaccinated. Although not focused on cancer, it can be seen how the direct engagement of the general population in research and audit can rapidly provide useful data.

An example of rapid data collection, sharing and collaboration from within cancer care would be the UK Coronavirus Cancer Monitoring Project (UKCCMP). This was established in March 2020 in the United Kingdom, the project rapidly recruiting groups of oncology doctors at 90% of UK cancer centres. These physicians collected, and reported, clinical data from patients with a cancer diagnosis who contracted SARS-CoV-2 infection. By using this methodology, a relatively large cohort of patients could be rapidly analysed in a short time. By May 2020, the project had amassed data on 1044 patients with a cancer diagnosis who also had COVID-19. On publication, this research was able to demonstrate the relatively high risk of mortality from COVID-19 in patients with a haematological malignancy in comparison to those with a solid tumour [3]. There are similar studies to this from other countries employing similar methodologies.

'Big Data' has been defined as 'a term describing the storage and analysis of large and/or complex data sets….' [4]. In some cases, this data can be collected prospectively with a specific research project in mind; in other cases, this data is collected for a range of different purposes but could then be used in research projects. An example of the latter is the use of DATA-CAN data to analyse the effect of the COVID-19 pandemic on cancer services and cancer patients in the United Kingdom during the first lockdown. DATA-CAN is the UK's Health Data Research Hub for Cancer and collects information from national health service (NHS) organisations, patients, charities, academia and industry. The researchers used real-time data collected during the pandemic and compared it with data pre-COVID-19. This showed a significant drop in urgent referrals for early cancer diagnosis and a reduction in chemotherapy attendances during the first wave of the pandemic. The results showed a real, rather than anecdotal, impact on cancer services with patients not wishing to report symptoms, attend their general practitioner (GP) or attend hospital [5]. These findings were reported to the UK government, and this resulted in a campaign to urge people to see their GP if they had cancer symptoms and highlight the importance of early diagnosis and attending hospital appointments [6].

In terms of research methodology, the ability to collect and share large quantities of real-time data from a range of sources (including direct reporting from research subjects) and store this in a form able to be analysed quickly has revolutionised public health research and allowed a rapid and coordinated response to the pandemic.

Telehealth and Virtual Consultations

Telehealth is defined by the Telehealth Resource Centre as 'A collection of means or methods for enhancing the healthcare, public health, and health education delivery and support using telecommunications technologies'. [1] In many ways, the widespread employment of non-face-to-face appointments for patients was the biggest change experienced by clinicians working in cancer care over the course of the pandemic. Internationally, the use of video conferencing, telephone and email consultations has increased dramatically [7]. The telephone appears to be the most widely used technology in telehealth across the world, but in the USA, the use of video conferencing is employed more widely than elsewhere [8]. The training required to provide effective delivery of virtual consultations and the effect on the patient experience will be specifically considered in later chapters (see Chap. 5).

There is an obvious need to provide guidelines to health professionals when using telemedicine. A key part of the process would be the need to obtain informed consent as it is important to point out associated risks that which may occur as a consequence of using telemedicine. Figure 4.1 illustrates how this consent can be integrated into an overarching process (see Fig. 4.1).

(a) **Telephone Consultations.** The telephone has been used in oncology appointments as an alternative to face-to-face consultation for many years. For example, the use of telephone review in patients receiving chemotherapy is well established and is used by doctors and allied health professionals to consult with patients, check general health post chemotherapy and, in some cases, allow for the next cycle of or dose of systemic anti-cancer treatment (SACT) to be safely delivered [10]. It is also used extensively as a tool to assess patients formally (via triage helplines) or informally, for example, by specialist nurses contacting patients in the community. The telephone is a widely used and available technology and is a flexible alternative to bringing patients into a healthcare environment. The limitations of the technology do not allow for visual assessment of the patient, reduce the effectiveness of communication by the

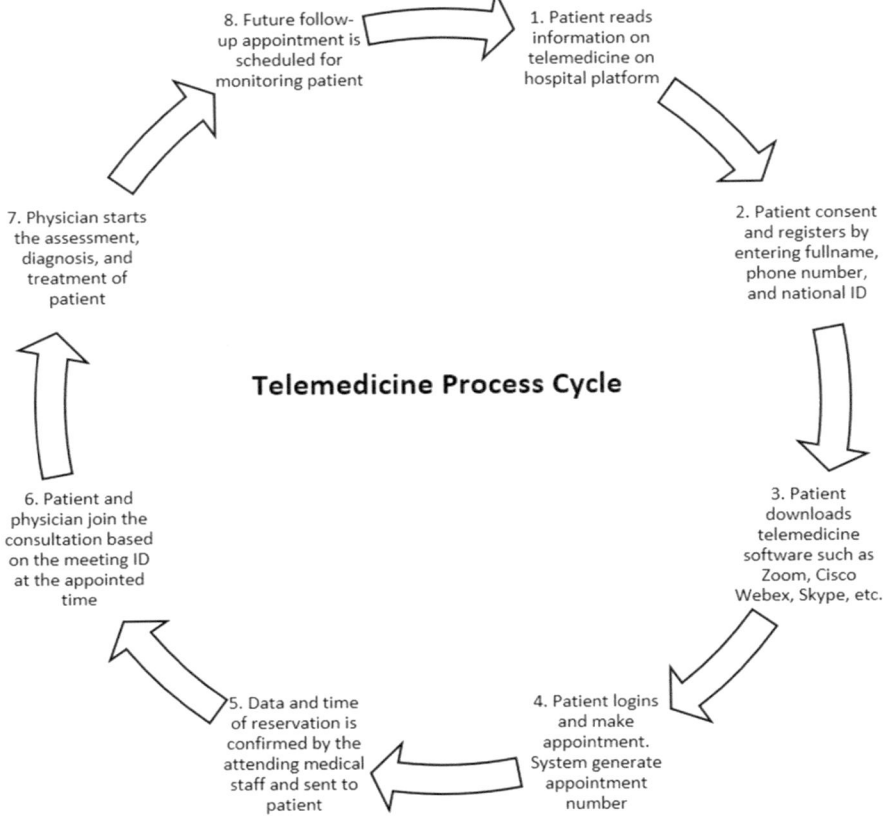

Fig. 4.1 The telemedicine process life cycle (This article is licensed under a Creative Commons Attribution 4.0 International License) [9]

absence of non-verbal cues and definitely do not allow any examination of the patient or physical assessment. To some extent, these shortfalls can be addressed by focused training on those using the telephone to assess patients.

(b) **Video Conferencing.** Video conferencing technology has been utilised in healthcare for some years, but this has been typically focused on education and the delivery of clinical meetings. Oncology centres were already developing video technology in order to prevent patients from travelling long distances to meet healthcare professionals, particularly in supportive care [11]. However, the huge change during the pandemic has been the much more widespread employment of this technology in clinical consultations with patients. There was increasing interest in the use of video conferencing technology with patients prior to the COVID-19 pandemic, with calls for more reliable evidence [12], but the pandemic provided a galvanising and urgent requirement to move to non-face-to-face forms of consultation. Across Europe, the rapid deployment of video conferencing technology has been variable between, and within, health systems. The deployment has been dependent on the availability of usable hardware, the ability and flexibility of healthcare settings to use existing software, the ability to develop and utilise health-specific software and the ability of specific populations of people with cancer to access both hardware and software. The long-term effects on healthcare delivery, both positive and negative, have yet to be fully realised and will be discussed later in this chapter. There are real concerns that sections of communities may well be significantly disadvantaged by the use of this type of technology particularly those with limited access to computers, a poor grasp of the language used by the healthcare professional in the consultation or a general lack of confidence with technology. These disadvantaged groups may include those defined by increased age, race/ethnicity and living in rural versus urban areas [13].

Changes to Education, Sharing Research and Conferencing

The delivery of effective and evidence-based cancer care in the United Kingdom and Europe is dependent on the ability to educate healthcare professionals and to share research and best practice. The COVID-19 pandemic has had a huge impact on the ability to do this. The effect on educating healthcare professionals will be considered in detail in Chap. 8, but suffice it to say that the move to deliver increasing elements of education virtually or 'online' became a necessity during the pandemic with all in-classroom and face-to-face lectures ceasing across Europe and the United Kingdom. In addition to these many clinical placements, a cornerstone of most clinical courses was also cancelled. Sometimes this has been because of concerns about transmitting coronavirus between different groups of staff but, certainly during the first wave and occasionally during subsequent waves, because the students had been deployed to support clinical areas. In their editorial written during the first wave of the pandemic, Swift et al. (2020) [14] described nursing students from year two of their degree programme in the United Kingdom onwards; they were asked to opt in to an extended placement working to boost the numbers of care staff available. As the pandemic has become more predictable, clinical placements recommenced but with increasing interest in carrying these out in a more controlled environment. To this end, 'virtual placements' have been trialled such as the peer-enhanced e-placements (PEEP model) in occupational therapy courses. These innovations are likely to be further extended into training for other healthcare professionals (see further reading).

The dissemination of research and best practice is vital in oncology, and one of the major means of bringing this about has been attending, and presenting at, conferences. There has been a network of large oncology conferences across the United Kingdom and Europe for many years, and these occur typically in large cities with good transport links. These can either be of general interest with sessions focused on particular tumour sites or aspects of care, or smaller site-specific conferences (such as in lung or breast cancer). These are largely medically driven events, but are often accompanied by sessions, or even whole programmes, which are of interest to oncology nurses or other members of the healthcare team. Conferences are typically funded via sponsorship by pharmaceutical companies or other companies involved in healthcare. A good example of this type of conference is the annual European Society for Medical Oncology (ESMO) conference which is run concurrently with the annual European Oncology Nursing Society (EONS) meeting. This provides a huge hub for oncologists, oncology nurses and sponsors to gather, network and share the latest research in the form of oral presentations or posters. It is one of the largest oncology conferences in the world with an attendance of around 25,000. Each country also has a network of smaller oncology conferences with some site specialism and some specialised by occupation. This system of in-person conferences was in effect, completely dismantled by the pandemic with virtually all events cancelled in both 2020 and 2021. In place of these conferences, there arose a series of virtual events with either pre-recorded or live presentations and with attendees 'logging on' to experience these. During the pandemic, this type of virtual education provided the only way for professionals to be informed of new developments, i.e. drugs, in a sharing environment, which allowed for discussion.

Despite the urgent manner in which these events were established, it quickly became apparent that a new model had emerged for delivering conferencing. This new type of oncology conference is certainly friendlier to the environment as they require no travel. There is no travelling time and hence no travelling budget; the sessions could be accessed from the clinical environments in which attendees worked and could be fitted around their other responsibilities. Could it be that the model of face-to-face conference is no longer relevant in the post-pandemic era? As some traditional conferences return in 2022, this largely remains to be seen, but Dr. David Oliver writing eloquently in the *British Medical Journal* discussed the pros and cons of physically attending large conferences and in the end produced a persuasive piece about their benefits [15]. In the online version, the possibilities for networking are very much reduced, the ability to discuss posters and presentations with the people who produce them is also reduced, and attending online, he argued, is a much less enriching experience than attending in person. The online conference may actually be a less effective way of sharing research and best practice. In the final analysis, it might be that the final arbiter of whether online conferences remain in place over traditional conference formats is the degree to which they can be sponsored by large pharmaceutical companies and other healthcare industries.

Despite the, now ubiquitous, nature of online conferencing, there is little comparative work to suggest how effective the format might be. In work that predates the pandemic, Maria Jose Sa and her fellow researchers [16] conducted a literature review and found that the virtual format may enhance academic participation, reducing some inequalities resulting from factors such as gender, race/ethnicity or social class but indicated that a hybrid approach combining both in-person and virtual elements might fulfil the needs of a majority of stakeholders. They may also offer more opportunities for unfunded professionals to attend as they are cheaper and cost much less time and financial resources to attend. The hybrid approach to conferencing is a new one, and the methodologies are in their relative infancy.

Outside of oncology, Puccinelli et al. [17] considered the challenges and comparative advantages and disadvantages of running hybrid conferences. The conclusions reached were that hybrid conferences offered a higher level of flexibility to participants as online-only event cannot replace the direct interactions present in an in-person event. They also recognised, however, that hybrid conferences are currently more expensive to run in comparison to both in-person and online-only events.

Technologically Delivered Therapeutic Interventions in Oncology

Accompanying the move to utilise technology to consult with patients and colleagues, there has been an increased interest and activity in delivering therapeutic interventions via similar routes. These interventions could be delivered via telephone, video software (either in person or pre-recorded) or via bespoke applications on mobile phones or wearable devices. For the purposes of this review, therapeutic interventions can be defined as being non-pharmacological in nature and capable of being replicated and delivered to patients or carers and potentially capable of delivering benefit.

The telephone offers the most straightforward and easily accessible way to deliver clinical interventions in a non-face-to-face format. A Cochrane review was published in 2020 [18] considering evidence for the effectiveness of telephone-delivered interventions in reducing symptoms associated with cancer and its treatment. The authors found some evidence supporting the use of telephone-delivered interventions for symptom management for adults with cancer. The studies included in the review predated the pandemic. The researchers also found that many of the studies were small and tended to vary widely in terms of methodology and called for 'robust and adequately reported trials …. across all cancer-related symptoms…or at the very least efforts should be made to standardise outcome measures'. With increased focus on not bringing patients into healthcare environments unless absolutely necessary, there may be renewed interest in providing robust evidence for telephone-delivered interventions in oncology; in any case, the use of the telephone to deliver therapeutic interventions is likely to continue.

The use of video technology or personal conferencing software to deliver therapeutic interventions has been employed much more extensively across the United Kingdom and Europe during the pandemic period. There are particularly high levels of interest and activity in employing this technology to promote physical activity and provide complementary or integrative therapies and psychological support programmes.

In recent years, there has been an acknowledgement that increased levels of physical activity can promote improved outcomes and quality of life in people with a cancer diagnosis [19–20] and health systems have begun to promote physical activity in this patient group. As the pandemic closed down in-person exercise classes or face-to-face promotion or management of programmes, where possible, these systems then relied on technology to deliver these. Telephone interaction is not immediately a format that translates to oversight or demonstration of physical activity, but video can be employed in this way. There appears to be considerable evidence, albeit from a range of small studies, that group classes delivered by video improved attendance and long-term adherence without any increased risk although, in some groups, barriers to participation existed in access to and the ability to use and adapt to the technology [21–22].

The provision of complementary therapies alongside traditional clinical treatments has increased widely across the United Kingdom and Europe over the last 15 years with many international studies reporting a beneficial effect of these on patient experience, reducing anxiety and improving mental health outcomes and managing symptoms (see recommended reading). The COVID-19 pandemic curtailed all non-essential physical contact and face-to-face interaction between healthcare providers and patients. Complementary therapies were particularly badly affected by this, being unrelated to the delivery of direct clinical therapies such as SACT or radiotherapy. In most cases, complementary therapies have also been slower to return to clinical environments for the same reason. An additional impact is that therapists delivering complementary therapies are much more likely to be independent practitioners and not directly employed by healthcare providers and therefore suffered a substantial financial impact. A Norwegian study [23] found considerable financial hardship with many therapists spending savings, relying on other family members for money, taking out bank loans and being reliant on financial support from the state. A majority (62.7%) expressed uncertainty about the future of their practice. The same study found that more than half (57.4%) of the practitioners offered video consultations and 46.6% had telephone consultations. A further finding was that those therapists who had reorganised their practice to online consultations were more optimistic about the future.

Of course, not all complementary and integrative therapies can be delivered via telehealth methodologies, the most commonly offered being mindfulness and relaxation, both individually and in groups. The evidence for effectiveness in the virtual delivery of these techniques is somewhat limited given the recent and rapid deployment of these since 2020, but what evidence there is seems to suggest that they are both feasible and appealing to patients. [24–26]

Use of Digital Health Applications in Cancer Care in the COVID Age

In addition to the more straightforward use of technology to contact patients directly via the telephone or via video conferencing technology, the COVID-19 pandemic has seen expansion of the use of digital applications or 'apps' to monitor, report or engage in cancer care activity.

Digital applications were already widely used across Europe in oncology prior to the declaration of the COVID-19 pandemic in 2020. A Spanish study carried out in 2016 found 166 different digital applications used on smartphones related to cancer care [27]. These authors found that the applications mainly provided information, helped in diagnosing particular issues or were preventive in nature. Many applications had more than one purpose, but the biggest subgroup of applications (42) provided information about antineoplastic agents.

As we have seen, during the height of the pandemic, there was a reduction in the number of patients able to attend routine appointments in hospitals or in their normal healthcare providers in the community. Digital applications allow people with a cancer care diagnosis to access advice and information, report symptoms or other medical issues or even make contact with skilled practitioners at their normal providers or other practitioners outside of this.

There is little objective literature on appraising the use of digital applications in cancer care, but proceedings of two workshops from the USA would indicate that the COVID-19 epidemic has both accelerated the use of digital applications and proved a testing ground for these [28, 29]. It was broadly acknowledged that most applications rely on the patient-reported outcomes (PRO) for them to be effective. These PRO might broadly be defined as information about a person's health or well-being which is sourced directly from the individual. PRO used in applications might include symptoms, the scoring or self-assessment of physical or mental well-being or overall satisfaction with their care, or elements of it. There has been a recent recognition of the importance of PRO in oncology research, but cancer services have to be in a position to monitor PRO and respond appropriately. It may be that the structured use of digital applications will allow this to happen.

There are good and clear examples of individual digital applications making a positive contribution to patient care. Berry et al. (2014) carried out a random controlled trial on a digital self-care reporting tool and found that it reduced symptom distress in patients with various cancer diagnoses both during and after active cancer treatment [30]. A structured review of 66 studies found benefits to patients relating to symptom management, reduction in symptom distress, a decrease in unplanned hospitalisations and improved quality of life and survival [31].

Publications in the field also reference the need for digital applications to be integrated into the patient pathway, the need for proper assessment and building of evidence base and the requirement for regulation [2–31].

Implications of Extended Use of Telehealth in Cancer Care

The use of telehealth and digital technology allowed cancer care to continue to be delivered throughout the COVID-19 pandemic, albeit in a radically altered fashion. When reviewing the possible longer-term impact of technology, most commentors, in most countries throughout the world, believe that there will not be a wholesale return to the way in which care was delivered pre-pandemic. Most reviewers believe that the rapid adoption of telehealth has had many positive effects which extend beyond the end of the pandemic; in many cases, the changes that have occurred represent an acceleration of what was already in process. Many of these advantages are based around reduction in patient travel to healthcare environments, more efficient use of professional's time and overall convenience for healthcare providers. It is also important to note that the use of telehealth may offer the patient or client increased choice of a range of types of appointment or interaction.

Another issue worthy of consideration is that a move to a greater reliance on technology in healthcare would have to be accompanied by improved information security and improved cybersecurity. Prior to the COVID pandemic, large healthcare providers, such as the NHS in the United Kingdom, were the subject of cyber-attack and the deployment of malware in order to extort money. An example of this would be the very disruptive 'Wannacry' cyber-attack of 2017 which affected 60 organisations in the United Kingdom and then spread to a further 150 countries [32]. In the post-pandemic era, there has been an increased concern that healthcare is likely to be a main target for other cyber-attacks [33].

It is fair to say, however, that the evidence base for a move to a wholehearted embrace of the delivery of cancer care via telehealth and digital technology is not yet in place. Most commentators in this field are themselves healthcare professionals, and if we look at what evidence there is with regard to patient experience, then the picture is much less obvious.

Publication of audits of patients' experience with regard to the use of telehealth during the COVID pandemic generally finds that patients like the convenience of telephone and video consultations whilst recognising their limitations. More in-depth studies of the effectiveness of telehealth in cancer seem to suggest that these limitations are more marked when considering the more holistic elements of cancer care. Canadian research indicates that 'patients who received virtual care were less satisfied in the areas of emotional support, receiving resources and referrals and the involvement of family and friends in their care'. [34] Work carried out in Ireland concluded that 'while telephone and telemedicine appointments have been implemented to ensure public safety and protection, such models may not adequately address the complex supportive care needs of people living with and beyond cancer'. [35] This qualitative study found that telephone consultations added barriers to support and limited person-centeredness in care interactions. There are suggestions that the skills and training of the healthcare professionals carrying out the interaction and the extent to which they are familiar with the technology will influence how effective the interaction is [36].

It would be therefore interesting to consider the effect of increased use of telehealth on cancer nursing and specifically on the delivery of specialist cancer nursing (such as the work of clinical nurse specialists) whose functionality is based around the delivery of holistic patient-centred care and the assessment of psychosocial needs. Within the United Kingdom, there is considerable evidence that access to a cancer clinical nurse specialist has a range of positive effects on patient experience and care (see recommended reading), but there is not yet evidence considering how this role might be impacted by a wider adoption of telehealth by specialist cancer nurses.

Test Your Learning

Which areas of cancer care have been positively impacted by the adoption of digital technology and telehealth during the COVID-19 pandemic?
What evidence do you believe should be gathered before the use of this technology is extended?

References

1. Lonergan PE et al (2020) Rapid utilization of telehealth in a Comprehensive Cancer Center as a response to COVID-19: cross-sectional analysis. J Med Internet Res 22(7):e19322
2. Menni C et al (2022) COVID-19 vaccine waning and effectiveness and side-effects of boosters: a prospective community study from the ZOE COVID study. Lancet Infect Dis:1002–1010
3. Lee LYW, Cazier J-B, Starkey T et al (2020) COVID-19 prevalence and mortality in patients with cancer and the effect of primary tumour subtype and patient demographics: a prospective cohort study. Lancet Oncol 21:1309–1301
4. Ward JS, Barker A (2013) Undefined by data: a survey of big data definitions. arXiv preprint arXiv:1309.5821
5. Lai AG, Pasea L, Banerjee A et al (2020) Estimated impact of the COVID-19 pandemic on cancer services and excess 1-year mortality in people with cancer and multimorbidity: near real-time data on cancer care, cancer deaths and a population-based cohort study. BMJ Open 10:e043828. https://doi.org/10.1136/bmjopen-2020-0438287
6. Macmillan cancer Support (2020) 'The Forgotten 'C'? The impact of Covid-19 on cancer care' published October 2020. Available at https://www.macmillan.org.uk/dfsmedia/1a6f23537f7f4519bb0cf14c45b2a629/9601-10061/the-forgotten-c-the-impact-of-covid-on-cancer-care. Last Accessed Feb 2023
7. Webster P (2020) Virtual health care in the era of COVID-19. Lancet 395:1180–1181
8. Loree JM, Dau H, Rebić N, Howren A, Gastonguay L, McTaggart-Cowan H, Gill S, Raghav K, De Vera MA (2021) Virtual oncology appointments during the initial wave of the COVID-19 pandemic: an international survey of patient perspectives. Curr Oncol 28(1):671–677. https://doi.org/10.3390/curroncol28010065
9. Bokolo A (2020) Use of telemedicine and virtual Care for Remote Treatment in response to COVID-19 pandemic. J Med Sys 44(7):132
10. Upton J (2016) Nurse-led telephone assessments for patients receiving ipilimumab. Cancer Nursing Pract 15(2)
11. Worster B, Swartz K (2017) Telemedicine and palliative care: an increasing role in supportive oncology. Curr Oncol Rep 19:37
12. Greenhalgh T et al (2016) Virtual online consultations: advantages and limitations (VOCAL) study. BMJ Open 6:e009388. https://doi.org/10.1136/bmjopen-2015-009388
13. Jewett PI, Vogel RI, Ghebre R et al (2022) Telehealth in cancer care during COVID-19: disparities by age, race/ethnicity, and resi (dential) status). J Cancer Surviv 16:44–51
14. Swift A et al (2020) COVID-19 and student nurses: a view from England. J Clin Nurs 00:1–4
15. Oliver D (2022) Has covid killed the medical conference? BMJ 376:o412. https://doi.org/10.1136/bmj.o412
16. Sa MJ, Ferreira CM, Serpa S (2019) Virtual and face-to-face academic conferences: comparison and potentials. J Edu Soc Res 9(2):35–47
17. Puccinelli E et al (2022) Hybrid conferences: opportunities, challenges and ways forward. bioRxiv:2022.03.18.484941. https://doi.org/10.1101/2022.03.18.484941

18. Ream E, Hughes AE, Cox A, Skarparis K, Richardson A, Pedersen VH, Wiseman T, Forbes A, Bryant A (2020) Telephone interventions for symptom management in adults with cancer. Cochrane Database Syst Rev (6):CD007568. https://doi.org/10.1002/14651858.CD007568.pub2. Last Accessed 12 Apr 2022
19. Patel AV et al (2019) American college of sports medicine roundtable report on physical activity, sedentary behavior, and cancer prevention and control. Med Sci Sports Exerc 51(11):2391–2402. https://doi.org/10.1249/MSS.0000000000002117
20. Friedenreich CM, Stone CR, Cheung WY, Hayes SC (2020) Physical activity and mortality in cancer survivors: a systematic review and meta-analysis. JNCI Cancer Spectrum 4(1). https://doi.org/10.1093/jncics/pkz080
21. Winters-Stone KM, Boisvert C, Li F et al (2022) Delivering exercise medicine to cancer survivors: has COVID-19 shifted the landscape for how and who can be reached with supervised group exercise? Support Care Cancer 30:1903–1906. https://doi.org/10.1007/s00520-021-06669-w
22. Pringle A, Kime N, Zwolinsky S, Rutherford Z, Roscoe CMP (2022) An investigation into the physical activity experiences of people living with and beyond cancer during the COVID-19 pandemic. Int J Environ Res Public Health 19(5):2945. https://doi.org/10.3390/ijerph19052945
23. Stub T, Jong MC, Kristofferson AE (2021) The impact of COVID-19 on complementary and alternative medicine providers: a cross-sectional survey in Norway' advances. Integrat Med 8:247–255
24. Knoerl R, Phillips CS, Berfield J et al (2021) Lessons learned from the delivery of virtual integrative oncology interventions in clinical practice and research during the COVID-19 pandemic. Support Care Cancer 29:4191–4194
25. Oh B, Van Der Saag D, Morgia M et al (2021) An innovative tai chi and Qigong telehealth Service in Supportive Cancer Care during the COVID-19 pandemic and beyond. Am J Lifestyle Med 15(4):475–477
26. Bailey-Dorton C, Yaguda S et al (2021) Rapid practice change during COVID-19 leads to enduring innovations and expansion of integrative oncology services. Oncology 36:26–32
27. Collado-Borrell R et al (2016) Smartphone applications for cancer patients; what we know about them? Farm Hosp 40(1)
28. National Academies of Sciences, Engineering, and Medicine (202) Opportunities and challenges for using digital health applications in oncology: proceedings of a workshop. The National Academies Press, Washington, DC. Available at http://nap.nationalacademies.org/26286. Last Accessed Feb 2023
29. Parikh RB et al (2022) Digital health applications in oncology: an opportunity to seize. J Natl Cancer Inst 114(10):djac108
30. Berry DL et al (2014) Electronic self-report assessment for cancer and self-care support: results of a multi-center randomized trial. J Clin Oncol 32:199–205
31. Aapro M, Bossi P, Dasari A et al (2021) Digital health for optimal supportive care in oncology: benefits, limits, and future perspectives. Support Care Cancer 28:4589–4612
32. Collier R (2017) NHS ransomware attack spreads worldwide. Can Med Assoc J 189(22):E786–E787
33. Kumar R, Sharma S, Vachhani C, Yadav N (2022) What changed in the cyber-security after COVID-19? Comput Secur 120:102821
34. Bultz B, Watson L (2021) Lessons learned about virtual cancer care and distress screening in the time of COVID-19'. Support Care Cancer 29:7535–7540
35. Drury A, Eicher M and Dowling M (2021) Experiences of cancer care during COVID-19: phase 1 results of a longitudinal qualitative study Int J Nursing Stud Adv 3, Pg 10030
36. Almathami HKY, Win KT, Vlahu-Gjorgievska E (2020) Barriers and facilitators that influence telemedicine-based, real-time, online consultation at patients homes: systematic literature review. J Med Internet Res 22(2)

Recommended Reading

Deng G (2019) Integrative medicine therapies for pain management in cancer patients. Cancer J (Sudbury, Mass.) 25(5):343–348

Gatellier L et al (2021) The impact of COVID-19 on cancer Care in the Post Pandemic World: five major lessons learnt from challenges and countermeasures of major Asian cancer Centres. Asian Pac J Cancer Prev 22(3):681–690

Kerr H, Donovan M, McSorley O (2021) Evaluation of the role of the clinical nurse specialist in cancer care: an integrative literature review. Eur J Cancer Care 30(3)

Lombe D, Sullivan R et al (2021) Silver linings: a qualitative study of desirable changes to cancer care during the COVID-19 pandemic. eCancer **15**:1202

Lyman GH et al (2018) Integrative therapies during and after breast cancer treatment: ASCO endorsement of the SIO clinical practice guideline. J Clin Oncol 36(25):2647–2265

Saleh A et al (2021) Being assigned a clinical nurse specialist is associated with better experiences of cancer care: English population-based study using the linked National Cancer Patient Experience Survey and cancer registration dataset. Eur J Cancer Care 30(6)

Taylor L (2020) Clinical placements: online options for learning during COVID-19 and beyond. Available at https://rcni.com/nursing-standard/students/nursing-studies/clinical-placements-online-options-learning-during-covid-19-and-beyond-169581. Last Accessed April 2022

Open Access This chapter is licensed under the terms of the Creative Commons Attribution 4.0 International License (http://creativecommons.org/licenses/by/4.0/), which permits use, sharing, adaptation, distribution and reproduction in any medium or format, as long as you give appropriate credit to the original author(s) and the source, provide a link to the Creative Commons license and indicate if changes were made.

The images or other third party material in this chapter are included in the chapter's Creative Commons license, unless indicated otherwise in a credit line to the material. If material is not included in the chapter's Creative Commons license and your intended use is not permitted by statutory regulation or exceeds the permitted use, you will need to obtain permission directly from the copyright holder.

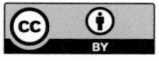

Virtual Consultations: Considering Staff Training and Patient Experience

Catherine Oakley and Emma Rowland

Introduction

As we see elsewhere in this publication, the early days of the COVID-19 pandemic forced rapid decision-making to address patient-safety concerns and maximise capacity in hospitals across Europe. The COVID-19 pandemic resulted in a huge increase in virtual consultations, particularly for cancer treatment appointments and generally without methodological processes, so therefore lacked the evidence base to support from patient or system perspectives. However, patients appeared satisfied with telephone or virtual consultations during the COVID-19 pandemic [1]. In Spain, healthcare professionals found video consultations reduced hospital visits and were time efficient and preferable to phone calls because patients could be more safely assessed, but they also lacked personalisation. They were considered a better option for fitter patients not requiring examination [2].

Some patients, however, struggled with technology and access to the required equipment (e.g. smart devices and the Internet) [3, 4] risking inequitable healthcare [5]. For older adults, additional barriers included impaired hearing or cognitive function [1], and carers were required to support access [4]. Some clinicians also struggled and worried about technology, often switching to telephone where video consultations did not work well and/or were time-consuming [2, 4]

During the COVID-19 pandemic, video consultations generally worked well for patient education, including chemotherapy [4]. Prior to the pandemic, group pre-treatment systemic anti-cancer treatment (SACT) consultations were successfully

---

C. Oakley (✉)
Systemic Anti-Cancer Therapy Nurse Consultant, Guy's and St Thomas' NHS Foundation Trust, London, UK
e-mail: catherine.oakley2@nhs.net

E. Rowland
Division of Long-term conditions and Department of Child and Family Health, Faculty of Nursing, Midwifery and Palliative Care, King's College London, London, UK
e-mail: Emma.Rowland@kcl.ac.uk

© The Author(s) 2026
M. Foulkes et al. (eds.), *Cancer Care in the Post-COVID World*,
https://doi.org/10.1007/978-3-031-33855-7_5

implemented by following robust processes in two large UK cancer centres. Mount Vernon Cancer Centre in North London introduced a face-to-face group [6]. Patients found the group dynamic and supportive and felt able to ask questions and more able to cope with the treatment. Some expressed a preference for a 1:1 session as they did not want to discuss personal issues with others. A face-to-face SACT group established in Southampton [7] was moved to a virtual platform during the pandemic [8]. Both groups made good use of nurse time, and survey findings showed the majority of patients understood the treatment process and felt confident to manage the side effects. Some patients who attended the virtual group experienced technological difficulties or felt conversations were not easy. Digital resources that patients and their families could refer to anytime were also found to be useful during COVID-19 [9, 10]. Interestingly, prior to the COVID-19 pandemic, the addition of a chemotherapy information film to standard pre-treatment information resulted in increased confidence to report symptoms [11].

Preparing Patients for Anti-cancer Therapy (PrePACT) Project as an Example of a Planned and Sustainable Approach to Virtual Consultations

Prior to the commencement of the project at a large UK Cancer Centre, each patient attended a 1:1, one-hour nurse-led face-to-face pre-treatment consultation (PTC). There was a national shortage of SACT nurses, and the centre was struggling to resource the service (equating to 40 hours of nursing time each week) and wanted to look at other options, without compromising patient care or the SACT nursing experience. They also recognised the PTC is a complex intervention. Research suggests SACT pre-treatment information delivery may be ineffective due to patients' struggling to engage with high-volume, complex and frightening information [12–14]. Information delivery can heighten fears of dying from the cancer or SACT and a reluctance to self-care to manage or report side effects to acute oncology services (AOS) [14].

The preparing patients for anti-cancer therapy (PrePACT) group consultation project aimed to deliver a research-informed, high-quality family group PTC. The project team initially developed a research-based face-to-face group PTC and patient learning resource [15]. The COVID-19 pandemic expedited a move to deliver a fully digital model, including staff training, thus enabling patients and family members to join the pre-treatment sessions from different locations and reduce visits to the hospital.

The overall aims of the project were to develop a high-quality group PTC for patients and their families ensuring that they were psychologically and practically prepared and supported for SACT, to confidently manage symptoms and report these appropriately to AOS. In addition, the project aimed to equip nurses and support workers with the skills and confidence to deliver virtual group consultations. The project was divided into three phases:

- Phase 1: researching and understanding the potential effectiveness of group pre-treatment consultations (PTC) [15]
- Phase 2: developing and evaluating a face-to-face group PTC
- Phase 3: developing and evaluating a digital group PTC and staff training

Phase 1: Understanding Potential Effectiveness of Group Pre-treatment Consultations

The project team observed pre-treatment clinics where patients and families are given information about SACT by doctors and chemotherapy nurses. One-to-one qualitative interviews were conducted with patients and healthcare professionals as well as focus groups with patients, their families and chemotherapy nurses.

Patients told the team that the traditional information delivery style was overwhelming and hard to hear at a time when they were most frightened, before treatment started. Patients commented on extensive, rushed information with no time to absorb or think about questions. The nurses also noticed that the patients did not take the information in. Patients felt there was missing information, particularly about the emotional side of treatment. Some patients found the tour of the treatment suite a new and frightening experience. They felt unprepared for seeing other patients, who looked unwell, with no hair and attached to drips. This was a traumatic experience and a shock as reality dawned—they would be sitting in the chemotherapy chair soon. Chemotherapy nurses reported becoming fatigued by the emotional weight of up to five one-to-one PTCs in one day and often found they forgot what they had said to which patients. They considered one structured group session would be potentially better.

Phase 2: Developing and Evaluating a Group Pre-treatment Consultation

A group PTC was developed with patients and staff which focused on the patient agenda and engagement and discussion to get families working together. The aim was for patients and their families to feel psychologically and practically prepared and supported for SACT, to confidently manage symptoms and report these appropriately to AOS. The focus was on empowerment and normality (which is an important coping strategy for people with cancer) [16–18]. The model included strategies to enhance emotional and physical well-being, animations, patient experiencing postcards (How I got through…) and a few short films led by the experts (e.g. consultant, psychologist). There were case study-based interactive workshops, self-management information and a 'show-and-tell' of the patients' Cancer Research UK (CRUK) Your Cancer Treatment Record. Traffic light symptom reporting scenarios were included based on the UK Oncology Nursing Society (UKONS) symptom reporting tool as well as a virtual tour of the chemotherapy unit and a film about the cancer information service.

There were 11 face-to-face group PTCs held during 2019 with 33 patients about to start immunotherapy and 28 family members. Surveys were conducted with patients and family who attended a group as well as with those who attended the traditional 1:1 session.

A comparison of the group patient and family surveys, with those completed by patients and family members who attended 1:1 PTCs, showed the group session may be better at assisting patients and their families through:

- Reduced repetition from the doctor-led consent appointment
- Family feeling more able to support the patients through treatment
- Meeting more individual needs
- Increased confidence to manage normal life during treatment
- Increased confidence to manage symptoms
- Increased confidence in knowing when (severity of symptoms) to call AOS
- Greater awareness of the patient information and support service
- Providing a virtual rather than a face-to-face tour of the treatment suite

Phase 3: Developing and Evaluating a Digital Group Pre-reatment Consultation and Staff Training

The face-to-face groups were paused in 2020 due to the COVID-19 pandemic. The team trained the staff and reframed the sessions so that they could be delivered via a digital platform. Patients and staff reviewed and contributed to a patient e-learning resource content as this was developed and refined for both immunotherapy and chemotherapy sessions. The learning resource was expanded to include more short films with signposting to further information. Building on the patient story postcards, patients were filmed giving accounts of their experiences, top tips for coping during SACT and managing side effects. More films were made with the experts—e.g. physio- and cancer hair care. The group session continued to focus on discussion and engagement to get families working together to manage and report symptoms and the reinforcement of key messages, especially the reporting of symptoms. Patients made recommendations to adapt the content, and with their help, the team developed the e-learning resource for patients to work through prior to the group session, with signposting and as a reference throughout treatment.

A new support worker role was introduced to help patients with digital access. Staff training was identified as important in the second phase of the project, and online learning modules for nurses and support workers were developed. The training aimed to assist the nurses and support workers to enhance continuity of care and facilitate the development of stronger emotionally attached relationships with patients and their families [19]. This has been shown to reduce health professional's emotional labour, increase job satisfaction, reduce absenteeism due to fatigue and burnout and enhance their own emotional well-being so that they are more emotionally resilient and better prepared to support the patient and their family through their emotional journey [19–21].

The digital group sessions were launched in 2023, and 125 patients and family members attended during the first five months. Survey responses from 40 patients and 4 carers show 98% of attendees were overall satisfied with their experience of the online session. They found the sessions were generally well organised and supportive. They appreciated the e-learning resources and particularly liked the traffic light symptom reporting tool exercises (based on real case studies). This gave 91% of the patients confidence to call AOS if they were to become unwell. 91% of patients had viewed the e-learning resource ahead of the session, which facilitated group discussions. 100% of patients had the opportunity to ask questions and felt listened to. An 80% of patients felt able to discuss concerns about the treatment during the session, 89% felt confident to manage their side effects. Patients also appreciated the support of others in a similar position and the follow-up call with a nurse after the session to discuss any individual information or concerns.

Although they found the session useful, the findings are similar to others' work with group consultations in that not everyone felt comfortable sharing their feelings with others. Some struggled with the technology, to access teams and to use the functions such as the camera or microphone. There were 15 patients who declined to participate due to technical difficulties. The project team therefore introduced a weekly face-to-face group session, to give patients a choice of a virtual or face-to-face group.

Six of nine nurse facilitators completed a survey. All agreed that the online learning was pitched at the right level and that consultations went well. However, not everyone felt confident delivering the intervention, and 50% were asked a question by a patient or family member that they could not answer. Interviews with five nurses favoured face-to-face over digital sessions, citing better engagement and emotional connection. Technology could be challenging, with patients slow to join digital sessions even with support workers. New interactive communication skills training was introduced to enhance patient engagement, reduce information overload, manage difficult conversations and focus more on normal life, which is important to patients. A bespoke nursing guide was developed for telephone follow-up calls, which could become lengthy due to a focus on delivering side effect information (contained in the learning resource) rather than answering specific patient questions. A technological glitch affecting appointment invitations was resolved. Cover for the support worker was introduced as the group sessions did not run as smoothly when they were unavailable to prepare and support the patients to join the sessions.

The aim of PrePACT is to ensure all patients receive a holistic PTC and they are safely prepared to manage SACT treatments and side effects. The team ensure that patients with hearing, language or mental health issues or who lack Internet access that prevents them from joining a digital group are not disadvantaged. These patients are identified through referring clinicians. It was recognised that some older people may not have access to digital technology. A local survey of 440 cancer patients [22] found 87% had access to a digital device, but not all were confident in using this. Importantly, only 4% of cancer patients did not have any digital access. A key part of the support worker role is to optimise patient uptake. The team ensures all patients have access to the new intervention (learning resource and group session) at some level by:

1. Ensuring access to the learning resource (including films). The support worker helps patients with access to technology but who lack confidence in their ability to access the digital resource. Patients are helped to access the resource through their own device (possibly with support of family or friends). The team plan to also offer a supported session to access the learning resource at the cancer centre, also acting as a teaching session.
2. Ensuring access to the group session. The support worker optimises patients' ability to attend a group session (thus gaining the therapeutic benefits of experiencing the session alongside other patients). This is achieved by supporting patients to access the group remotely, including where required, practising joining the online platform and familiarisation with chat and raised hand functions.
3. Signposting patients to revisit the learning resource to help with symptom self-management. Patients, who lack digital access, can be offered an iPad on the treatment suite and helped to view the relevant side-effect sections of the learning resource. Importantly, the capacity created in chemotherapy nursing workload by the new support worker post will support the move to this model. The newly created capacity will enable a more enhanced level of support to be provided to patients for whom accessing the digital service is more difficult or not possible.

Implications for Digital Group PTC in Cancer Care

Group virtual consultations, if developed robustly, have the potential to save precious nursing resources and improve the experience of patients, family members and staff. The project team is also considering how this approach might be used for other groups of patients. For example, breast patient preoperative education sessions are often conducted individually (one patient/one nurse) where the same information is repeated to each patient.

The development and planning of PrePACT was established prior to the COVID-19 pandemic; however, the adaptations to the delivery of PrePACT from face-to-face to virtual consultations were a direct response to the COVID-19 pandemic and expansion of digital healthcare during this period. A coordinated and agile approach to the change, with strong leadership, enabled this intervention to be successful [4]. In addition, skills training in technological and communication is essential for healthcare professionals, and developing new roles to support patients with technology use is also required for the sustainability of digital patient care [2, 5].

Reviewing and drawing on the emerging evidence, co-design and ongoing evaluation and development of these types of interventions with patients and staff will be core to longevity and sustainability [23]. A particular focus of research should be on the implications and needs of more vulnerable patients who may struggle with technology, the best support worker, nursing model and potential for using artificial intelligence to make the information more easily updated and widely available to a diverse population. Such services should be carefully planned with a business case and associated training and digital resources.

Test Your Learning

How could patients, families and nurses benefit from switching from 1:1 to group PTC?

What would you need to include in a proposal for developing this type of service at your organisation?

References

1. Chen M et al (2022) Remaining agile in the COVID-19 pandemic healthcare landscape—how we adopted a hybrid telemedicine geriatric oncology care model in an academic tertiary cancer center. J Geriatr Oncol 13:856–861
2. Jiménez-Rodríguez D et al (2020) Increase in video consultations during the COVID-19 pandemic: healthcare professionals perceptions about their implementation and adequate management. Int J Environ Res Public Health 17:5112
3. Paterson C et al (2020) The role of telehealth during the COVID-19 pandemic across the interdisciplinary cancer team: implications for practice. Semin Oncol Nurs 36:151090
4. Mackwood M et al (2022) Adoption of telemedicine in a rural US cancer center amid the COVID-19 pandemic: qualitative study. JMIR Cancer 8:1–12
5. Bakitas M et al (2021) Telehealth strategies to support patients and families across the cancer trajectory. Am Soc Clin Oncol Educ B:413–422. https://doi.org/10.1200/EDBK_320979
6. Sullivan T, Harrold K, Bell K, Griffin C, Scarlett C (2013) Benefits of attending nurse-led pre-chemotherapy group sessions. Cancer Nurs Pract 12:27–31
7. Tomlins E, Fisher S, Gifford L, Weston A (2021) Evaluating group pre-assessment for improving self-efficacy in patients undergoing systemic anticancer therapy. Cancer Nurs Pract 20:36–42
8. Weston A (2022) Development of a digital pre-assessment pathway for patients starting systemic anticancer therapy. Cancer Nurs Pract 21:29–34
9. Turkdogan S et al (2021) Development of a digital patient education tool for patients with cancer during the COVID-19 pandemic. JMIR Cancer 7:1–6
10. Giuliani M, Papadakos T, Papadakos J (2020) Propelling a new era of patient education into practice—cancer care post–COVID-19. Int J Radiat Oncol Biol Phys 108:404–406
11. Kinnane N, Stuart E, Thompson L, Evans K, Schneider-Kolsky M (2008) Evaluation of the addition of video-based education for patients receiving standard pre-chemotherapy education. Eur J Cancer Care (Engl) 17:328–339
12. Treacy JT, Mayer DK (2000) Perspectives on cancer patient education. Semin Oncol Nurs 16:47–56
13. Skalla KA, Bakitas M, Furstenberg CT, Ahles T, Henderson JV (2004) Patients' need for information about cancer therapy. Oncol Nurs Forum 31:313–319
14. Oakley C et al (2017) Avoidant conversations about death by clinicians cause delays in reporting of neutropenic sepsis: grounded theory study. Psychooncology 26:1505–1512
15. Rowland E, Oakley C (2023) Exploring the acceptability and benefits of group pretreatment consultations for people receiving systemic anticancer therapy. Cancer Nurs Pract. https://doi.org/10.7748/cnp.2023.e1850
16. Strauss AL, Corbin J, Fagerhaugh S, Glaser BG, Maines D, Suczek B, Wiener C (1984) Chronic illness and the quality of life. Mosby Inc.

17. Cowley L, Heyman B, Stanton M, Milner SJ (2000) How women receiving adjuvant chemotherapy for breast cancer cope with their treatment: a risk management perspective. J Adv Nurs 31:314–321
18. Mitchell T (2007) The social and emotional toll of chemotherapy ? Patients' perspectives. Eur J Cancer Care (Engl) 16:39–47
19. Rowland E (2021) Case study 1: hospital-based multidisciplinary work—institutional emotional geographies. In: Andrews G, Rowland E, Peter E (eds) Place and professional practice: the geographies in health care work. Springer, pp 69–91. https://doi.org/10.1007/978-3-030-64179-5_3
20. Bolton SC (2004) Emotion management in the workplace. Bloomsbury Publishing Plc. https://doi.org/10.5040/9781350390751
21. Smith P (2012) The emotional labour of nursing revisited: can nurses still care? Palgrave Macmillian
22. Cotton A, Lavender V, Lei M (2022) Barriers to digital health in patients undergoing cancer treatment. In: UK Oncology Nursing Society (UKONS) conference, Belfast
23. Robert G et al (2022) Co-producing and co-designing. Cambridge University Press. https://doi.org/10.1017/9781009237024

Further Reading

Deng G (2019) Integrative medicine therapies for pain management in cancer patients. Cancer J (Sudbury, Mass.) 25(5):343–348

Open Access This chapter is licensed under the terms of the Creative Commons Attribution 4.0 International License (http://creativecommons.org/licenses/by/4.0/), which permits use, sharing, adaptation, distribution and reproduction in any medium or format, as long as you give appropriate credit to the original author(s) and the source, provide a link to the Creative Commons license and indicate if changes were made.

The images or other third party material in this chapter are included in the chapter's Creative Commons license, unless indicated otherwise in a credit line to the material. If material is not included in the chapter's Creative Commons license and your intended use is not permitted by statutory regulation or exceeds the permitted use, you will need to obtain permission directly from the copyright holder.

European Perspectives on Cancer and the Pandemic

6

Constantina Cloconi, Christina Alexopoulou, Nicole Zamba, Mary Economou, and Andreas Charalambous

Check your Knowledge and Experience
As European healthcare providers, what challenges did your healthcare system face during the severe acute respiratory syndrome coronavirus (SARS-CoV-2) pandemic?

What was the European perspective on cancer care during the SARS-CoV-2 pandemic?

Introduction

The healthcare systems around the world have faced a multitude of challenges during the severe acute respiratory syndrome coronavirus (SARS-CoV-2) pandemic over the past 2 years, from a number of aspects [1]. Although in the relevant literature, these have been primarily presented in isolation, for the purpose of this chapter, these have been grouped into categories. Organisational, psychological, socioeconomic challenges, as well as hindrances in continuing professional and scientific development, have undeniably affected the way in which healthcare

---

C. Cloconi
German Oncology Center/Cyprus University of Technology, Limassol, Cyprus
e-mail: constantina.cloconi@goc.com.cy

C. Alexopoulou · N. Zamba
German Oncology Center, Limassol, Cyprus
e-mail: Christina.Alexopoulou@goc.com.cy; Nicole.Zamba@goc.com.cy

M. Economou
Cyprus University of Technology, Limassol, Cyprus

A. Charalambous (✉)
Department of Nursing Science, Cyprus University of Technology, Limassol, Cyprus
e-mail: Andreas.charalambous@cut.ac.cy

© The Author(s) 2026
M. Foulkes et al. (eds.), *Cancer Care in the Post-COVID World*,
https://doi.org/10.1007/978-3-031-33855-7_6

professionals cared for patients, and it is worth taking the time to review how this was materialised.

Organisational Challenges

Healthcare Workforce

From an organisational perspective, infrastructural adaptations and the introduction of new hospital policies had a major impact on healthcare professionals, standard operating hospital procedures, outpatient visits and even family visitation rights of hospitalised patients. The most apparent impact the pandemic has had in this respect has to be on healthcare infrastructure. Major changes were implemented to medical buildings, in the form of facility expansions or repurposing existing spaces, to accommodate the heightened need for specialised units dedicated to patients with SARS-CoV-2. In turn, progressively more healthcare professionals were being transferred from their regular posts to such units, as demand continued to rise with increasing number of cases, leaving other wards understaffed and unable to efficiently carry out routine daily duties. Expectedly, healthcare professionals contracting the virus also contributed to staffing shortages which, along with a growing sick population, immensely overburdened health systems.

Inadequate staffing, however, was far from the only hurdle medical organisations had to circumvent. Hospitals across Europe were faced with the incredibly challenging task of maintaining functioning health services with a struggling workforce, medical supply shortages and an increasing demand for patient care.

Visitations and Medical Supply Shortages

The new practice standards and regulations that had been established in order to minimise transmission of the virus in hospital settings gave rise to an array of additional issues. With respect to bed availability, critically ill SARS-CoV-2 patients had flooded the wards, leaving close to no vacancy for admissions of any other nature. The high-speed consumption of resources and insufficient personnel made the management of chronic patients such as cancer patients, who are often immunocompromised and have complex symptomatology, increasingly more difficult [2, 3]. In addition, countless cancer patients that had contracted the virus had planned diagnostic tests and even treatments cancelled, increasing their risk of relapse, delayed treatment or even death. The findings of a study conducted in patients with head and neck cancer highlighted the importance of maintaining the care of cancer patients during the pandemic to reduce the risk of death due to delays [4]. Data released by the European Cancer Organisation as part of the "Time to Act" campaign [5] estimated that more than 100 million of screening tests have not been performed as a result of the pandemic. This resulted in an estimation of more than 1 million patients being undiagnosed with cancer. This has also created a significant backlog in these diagnostic tests, making it a challenging situation for healthcare systems to efficiently respond [5].

Along with the changes that had been made to patients' scheduled visits, appointments for diagnostic tests and treatments, new rules had also been enforced regarding hospital visitation rights. Patients were now expected to have their consultations and follow-up visits online, deviating from the contemporary norm, and family members could no longer visit their hospitalised relatives freely, frequently even denied the opportunity to say their final goodbyes [6]. The pandemic had also instilled a deep sense of alarm among the general public in visiting hospitals, which caused many to postpone or even entirely avoid going to their appointments in fear of contracting the virus [7, 8]. Though an understandable worry at a time when confronted with a disease that can potentially be fatal, especially in vulnerable groups, missed healthcare appointments were a particular concern for cancer patients. The unfortunate consequences for those who missed their appointments were interruptions in treatments, adversely affecting treatment outcomes owing to decreased local control and overall survival, not identifying early signs of relapse, leading to disease progression and delayed diagnosis of complications associated with their primary disease or even identification of secondary findings that cost many their lives [9]. In some countries, the lack of standardised telemedicine with informatic platforms caused various challenges. Furthermore, the need to rapidly introduce telemedicine services to patients resulted in various negative implications. For example, the typical model for direct-to-consumer telemedicine entails a single encounter between a clinician and patient who have no preceding relationship. The telemedicine approach prevents the clinician from the possibility to perform on-site testing, has no means to bring the patient in for a face-to-face examination and has little way to ensure the patient will access follow-up care if they get worse [10]. The implementation of specialist platforms for the teleassessment of cancer patients can grant patients' protection and improve the oncology pathways during crises (like SARS-CoV-2 pandemic) [11]. Effective telemedicine methods should recognise and take account of the challenges associated with physiological characteristics and the age of patients [12].

These organisational challenges, however, served as a seedbed for the development of new strategies to establish secure conditions in case of potential future crises. The introduction of specialised departments for communicable diseases in all hospitals is one example. During the pandemic, algorithms were also created to manage cancer patients requiring surgery, whether scheduled or emergency. Surgeries for those who had tested positive for the virus were postponed, if possible; otherwise, strict measures were taken to reduce postoperative complications and ensure both the safety of patients and healthcare professionals [3].

Socioeconomic

Crises of such magnitude as the SARS-CoV-2 pandemic affect all socioeconomic strata. Weakening of the social bond due to lockdowns, curfews, social distancing and other restrictive measures had profound negative effects on societies collectively around the globe. Patients from more deprived socioeconomic backgrounds, however, were especially affected, as those who suffered from cancer and the SARS-CoV-2 virus were forced to stop working but were not in turn offered appropriate social and economic support. Finding themselves in an even more vulnerable situation, some often experienced marginalisation and social stigmatisation. Their self-image suffered further as some felt they were not only physically excluded due to their illness and the accompanying changes it brought about in their bodies but also socially excluded due to the loss of their professional identity and any economic independence [13].

This is where the moral and ethical problem of using algorithms to prioritise the management of medical conditions arises. The principles of patient-centre care were significantly diminished as healthcare professionals were asked to triage patients according to predefined criteria, whatever they may be, when the ideal situation would be for everyone to be able to receive prompt and comprehensive medical care [14]. The very concept of triage is incompatible with the principle of providing adequate holistic care for each patient in accordance with their specific needs at any given moment. In a way, the use of algorithms may come to give a veneer of scientific or objective character to a categorisation of patients that is by definition contrary to the ethics of healthcare professionals who must care for all patients [15]. In a recent paper by Grote and Berens [16], it was argued that the deployment of such algorithms in healthcare not only challenges the epistemic authority of clinicians, but more importantly it somewhat promotes patterns of defensive decision-making which might come at the harm of patients. On the same topic, the SARS-CoV-2 pandemic has demonstrated how the strategy of 'first come, first served' should not apply in situations of emergency such as a pandemic. Although this appears to be legitimate as it might have a negative impact on resources (e.g. ICU) being withheld from a new patient because the bed is occupied by another patient who is predicted not to survive with a meaningful quality of life, it could be a more consequentialist perspective to care [17]. Based on such perspectives, there will be situations where the decision basis can be guided by supererogatory protocols, in which altruistic individuals are willing to renounce their ventilator to hand it over to (important/famous) patients who need it but cannot get it [18].

The question that arises, therefore, is to what extent can an algorithm be expected to address the ethical challenge posed by the inability to adequately care for all patients due to limited beds and staff?

Personal Challenges

Somatic Perspectives

Many healthcare professionals faced post-traumatic stress and long-term SARS-CoV-2 side effects. The disrupted work-life balance and limited resources were associated with higher levels of burnout due to longer shifts, stigma and the effects of SARS-CoV-2 infection itself [19, 20]. Healthcare professionals' levels of exhaustion were significantly elevated during the SARS-CoV-2 pandemic [21]. Compared to studies prior to the SARS-CoV-2 pandemic, these exhaustion levels were found to be significantly increased [22]. Healthcare professionals' most common side effects as a result of the inappropriate use of PPE during the long daily contacts with SARS-CoV-2 patients identified were fever, cough and weakness. Furthermore, skin damage and the nasal bridge were the most affected sites after prolonged use of PPE [23].

Psychological Perspective

Cancer patients are a particularly vulnerable group. For their safety, the measures put in place to combat the pandemic had, in turn, kept their families at a distance by limiting or even banning hospital visits [2]. These obstacles not only made it difficult to accompany terminally ill patients but also disrupted the process of mourning. Patients and their families were called to deal with these new circumstances, and as a result, some were lumbered with psychological issues.

Controlling behaviour exercised by healthcare professionals, health managers and policy makers, the desire to control everything in the name of new protection measures against the virus, the absence of equal conditions between private and public hospitals, appeared intrusive and frightening for the people who were already under maximum pressure. Health restrictions translated into isolation practices, where the effort to keep patients alive led to forms of psychological abuse.

Cancer patients experienced feelings of anxiety and depression. The modifications mentioned above concerning human contact, whether concerning outpatient visits to the doctor or relatives visiting their hospitalised family members, significantly affected anxiety levels [8].

In terms of social representations, the SARS-CoV-2 pandemic has been equated with an adversary or a battle, through a process of personification of the disease. This bellicose discourse, expressed in an aggressive way, has contributed to the polarisation of social practices, turning health restrictions into a privileged field for any form of abuse of power exercised against vulnerable or vulnerable individuals and groups. This was particularly true for the elderly, who were isolated in nursing homes for long periods of time, resulting in excessive and burdensome grief as a result of the restrictions to protect them from contracting SARS-CoV-2.

The measures taken have proved to be particularly detrimental to patients, their families and healthcare professionals, which has been the subject of all negative claims as the guardian of a provision perceived as inhumane. In other words, the strict application of the rules by medical staff contributed to a feeling of marginalisation, suffering and lack of understanding among patients and their families, who generally felt excluded from the support of their loved ones.

Sometimes this situation even led to families not being able to attend the funeral of their loved ones or burials with closed coffins. The inability to be present in the last moments of the lives of these loved ones, not feeling surrounded by the rest of the family and even not participating in the funeral ceremonies greatly complicated the process of mourning for many people [24].

This demonstrates the need to operate in a different way in future similar emergencies in order to provide the best possible support to patients and their families while maintaining an ethically acceptable position as healthcare professionals. With regard to the prospects of care and support, we therefore recommend maintaining visits to patients regardless of the health context, while of course observing all the necessary precautionary measures. This can be achieved by encouraging all forms of communication using technological means (mobile phones, computers or tablets) as mentioned in Chap. 4, 'Increasing Use of Technology in SARS-CoV-2 Pandemic and the Effect of This on Staff and Patients'.

This human contact through the new media should not hamper traditional ways of communication but should be added to the already existing means at our disposal. It is also up to the staff of the then hospital to supplement the approved visit time of the patients by offering a valuable presence to them and their relatives, even if nothing can replace the presence of the people we love (like videocalls) when we are very sick or at the end of our life [25, 26]. Activities should also be proposed to encourage the development of individual and interpersonal links. All artistic pursuits enhance the spirit of creativity. Combined with a group dimension, they can contribute to the emergence of new forms of sociability. Artistic pursuits such as painting, music or handicrafts can improve the feeling of isolation by leaving people to feel creative.

The aim of the medical institution may be to create a sense of protection, where the team of medical and paramedical staff help to create a protective envelope that supports the patient psychologically by helping them to cope with their deepest mental anguish.

It is extremely important for patients who are hospitalised to feel that the medical team is supportive of them and their creativity. Winnicott's studies show the importance of creativity as a process that allows the individual to work through their psychological struggles [27]. Creativity is a form of alchemy that entails the transformation of mourning and loss into a process of psychological healing which is proven to be valuable to patients [28].

The pandemic has highlighted the need to create protocols that take into account the human factor. For example, during the pandemic, healthcare professionals' main goal was to prevent the transmission of the virus by isolating healthcare workers, patients and families, without taking into account their personal needs. Protection against the virus was paramount. The findings of a study conducted on healthcare professionals dealing with cancer patients showed significant levels of burnout, reduced coping capacities and decreased resilience among cancer care professionals. This study highlights the need for timely and appropriate preparation of healthcare systems to better support professionals involved in the care of cancer patients, in case of a new SARS-CoV-2-type emergency. So, if we want to adequately support healthcare professionals, it is advisable to train them by taking into account all three factors mentioned, so that they are ready to manage such situations, having acquired coping and resilience skills in conditions that favour burnout [19].

Perspectives in Continuing Professional and Scientific Development

Improving and advancing our knowledge at the time of the SARS-CoV-2 pandemic has proven to be quite difficult. The exchange of ideas and new practices for the better care of cancer patients had taken another form with the transition to online courses, webinars and other virtual workshops. The resulting lack of in-person interactions largely contributed to the reduced effectiveness of such learning events. It is also important to note the effects of the pandemic on the conduct of clinical studies. Clinical studies during the pandemic showed an increase in protocol deviations, delays were observed and funding interruptions occurred due to the global financial situation. All efforts in research were directed towards the development of vaccines against the emerging coronavirus, hence deprioritising most other research studies [2, 29].

Ethical issues affect the very conduct of clinical trials, as they are often influenced by economic considerations and thus heavily dependent on the strategic priorities of the companies funding them. Pandemic circumstances have disrupted the way trials are conducted; therefore, new methods have been developed and adopted more widely to facilitate recruitment, consent and overall trial conduct. The question that arises is to what extent the individual needs of groups of patients or of each individual patient are taken into account in light of these changes in the design and implementation of clinical trials. For example, in a study by He et al. [30], 3765 COVID-19 clinical study summaries that were downloaded from the *ClinicalTrials.gov* trial registry were analysed. The analyses demonstrated that specific groups of patients were systematically excluded such as pregnant women. The same study reported that known risk factors such as diabetes, hypertension, obesity and asthma, which may lead to serious illnesses, were considered by less than 5% of the studies that were reviewed.

Conclusion

The experience of the pandemic has brought new perspectives on health and particularly on cancer. The unprecedented conditions created by the pandemic forced the healthcare systems, healthcare professionals, patients and the public to effectively and efficiently adjust to.

The high transmissibility of the virus, coupled with stringent restrictions on physical contact, has facilitated the widespread adoption of teleconsultations as a strategy to minimize hospital visits and mitigate the risk of viral transmission, particularly among vulnerable populations such as cancer patients.

In addition, the need for further education and training for healthcare professionals on crises' management such as the pandemic SARS-CoV-2 seemed to emerge. Despite previous experiences with the outbreaks of the Middle East respiratory syndrome coronavirus (MERS-CoV) and severe acute respiratory syndrome (SARS), the scale of the SARS-CoV-2 has challenged the preparedness and resilience of healthcare systems around the world. Maintaining the provision of quality care requires high-level and ongoing training for healthcare professionals. This is deemed necessary to continue the provision of routine care to patients but also caring for those who contract the virus resulting in additional physical, psychological and social needs. Putting in place crisis-management protocols is essential to safeguard the resilience of the healthcare professionals and the healthcare organisations overall. Furthermore, the development of programmes to manage burnout and stress is also necessary since during the pandemic issues such as stigma, social isolation, shortages and working conditions were conducive to their increase. A report [31] on how countries have supported their health workers in 36 countries in Europe and Canada has revealed numerous initiatives taken based on data extracted from the COVID-19 Health Systems Response Monitor (HSRM). With reference to supporting the mental health of their healthcare workers, most countries in Europe (e.g. Bulgaria, Czech Republic, France, Malta, Romania) have established helplines that health and oftentimes social care workers can call to access psychological support from trained professionals [31].

Finally, the value of multidisciplinary teams was highlighted during the pandemic. These teams allowed for the exchange of ideas resulting in innovative solutions to managing the many challenges posed by the pandemic both at an organisational and at a personal level. Such collaborations present a pivotal way to cultivating a resilience culture within the context of healthcare organisations. A mixed methods study [32] that was undertaken among a large sample of healthcare employees in Switzerland focused on problematic real-world situations experienced by them and their managers during the pandemic's first wave. The study highlighted the importance of the need and importance of meso-level adaptations adopted by institutions and micro-level strategies put in place by teams and employees. With respect to the latter, strategies that were implemented to support the better functioning and well-being of the multidisciplinary team, such as in terms of communication skills, cooperation, decision making, conflict resolution and emotional burdens, have contributed to the increase of their resilience.

Test your Learning
What is the impact of the pandemic on healthcare professionals?
What changes do you believe are required to effectively face the healthcare system's challenges posed by future pandemics?

Conflict of Interest The authors don't have any conflict of interest to declare.

References

1. Gultekin M, Ak S, Ayhan A, Strojna A, Pletnev A, Fagotti A, Perrone AM, Erzeneoglu BE, Temiz BE, Lemley B, Soyak B, Hughes C, Cibula D, Haidopoulos D, Brennan D, Cola E, van der Steen-Banasik E, Urkmez E, Akilli H et al (2021) Perspectives, fears and expectations of patients with gynaecological cancers during the COVID-19 pandemic: a Pan-European study

of the European Network of Gynaecological Cancer Advocacy roups (ENGAGe). Cancer Med 10(1):208–219. https://doi.org/10.1002/cam4.3605
2. Gasper H, Ahern E, Roberts N, Chan B, Lwin Z (2020) COVID-19 and the cancer care workforce: from doctors to ancillary staff. Semin Oncol 47(5):309–311. https://doi.org/10.1053/j.seminoncol.2020.06.001
3. Hwang ES, Balch CM, Balch GC, Feldman SM, Golshan M, Grobmyer SR, Libutti SK, Margenthaler JA, Sasidhar M, Turaga KK, Wong SL, McMasters KM, Tanabe KK (2020) Surgical oncologists and the COVID-19 pandemic: guiding cancer patients effectively through turbulence and change. Ann Surg Oncol 27(8):2600–2613. https://doi.org/10.1245/s10434-020-08673-6
4. Matos LL, Forster CHQ, Marta GN, Castro Junior G, Ridge JA, Hirata D, Miranda-Filho A, Hosny A, Sanabria A, Gregoire V, Patel SG, Fagan JJ, D'Cruz AK, Licitra L, Mehanna H, Hao SP, Psyrri A, Porceddu S, Galloway TJ et al (2021) The hidden curve behind COVID-19 outbreak: the impact of delay in treatment initiation in cancer patients and how to mitigate the additional risk of dying—the head and neck cancer model. Cancer Causes Control 32(5):459–471. https://doi.org/10.1007/s10552-021-01411-7
5. European Cancer Organisation (2022) Time to act campaign. https://www.europeancancer.org/timetoact
6. Gao Z, Yang Y, Ding C, Niu P, Huang W, Lei F, Gu J (2020) Oncologists' perspective: when cancer encounters COVID-19. Oncologist 25(9):e1423–e1423. https://doi.org/10.1634/theoncologist.2020-0296
7. Manso L, de Velasco G, Paz-Ares L (2020) Impact of the COVID-19 outbreak on cancer patient flow and management: experience from a large university hospital in Spain. ESMO Open 5(3). https://doi.org/10.1136/esmoopen-2020-000828
8. Momenimovahed Z, Salehiniya H, Hadavandsiri F, Allahqoli L, Günther V, Alkatout I (2021) Psychological distress among cancer patients during COVID-19 pandemic in the world: a systematic review. Front Psychol 12. https://doi.org/10.3389/fpsyg.2021.682154
9. Thomson CA, Overholser LS, Hébert JR, Risendal BC, Morrato EH, Wheeler SB (2021) Addressing cancer survivorship care under COVID-19: perspectives from the cancer prevention and control research network. Am J Prev Med 60(5):732–736. https://doi.org/10.1016/j.amepre.2020.12.007
10. Shaver J (2022) The state of telehealth before and after the COVID-19 pandemic. Prim Care 49(4):517–530. https://doi.org/10.1016/j.pop.2022.04.002
11. Indini A, Pinotti G, Artioli F, Aschele C, Bernardi D, Butera A, Defraia E, Fasola G, Gamucci T, Giordano M, Iaria A, Leo S, Ribecco AS, Rossetti R, Savastano C, Schena M, Silva RR, Grossi F, Blasi L (2021) Management of patients with cancer during the COVID-19 pandemic: the Italian perspective on the second wave. Eur J Cancer 148:112–116. https://doi.org/10.1016/j.ejca.2021.01.040
12. López-Fernández A, Villacampa G, Grau E, Salinas M, Darder E, Carrasco E, Torres-Esquius S, Iglesias S, Solanes A, Gadea N, Velasco A, Urgell G, Torres M, Tuset N, Brunet J, Corbella S, Balmaña J (2021) Patients' and professionals' perspective of non-in-person visits in hereditary cancer: predictors and impact of the COVID-19 pandemic. Genet Med 23(8):1450–1457. https://doi.org/10.1038/s41436-021-01157-2
13. Zeilinger EL, Knefel M, Schneckenreiter C, Pietschnig J, Lubowitzki S, Unseld M, Füreder T, Bartsch R, Masel EK, Adamidis F, Kum L, Kiesewetter B, Zöchbauer-Müller S, Raderer M, Krauth MT, Staber PB, Valent P, Gaiger A (n.d.) The impact of COVID-19 and socioeconomic status on psychological distress in cancer patients. https://doi.org/10.1101/2022.11.21.22282580
14. Petrini C (2010) Triage in public health emergencies: ethical issues. Intern Emerg Med 5(2):137–144. https://doi.org/10.1007/s11739-010-0362-0
15. Kuipers SJ, Nieboer AP, Cramm JM (2021) Making care more patient centered; experiences of healthcare professionals and patients with multimorbidity in the primary care setting. BMC Fam Pract 22(1). https://doi.org/10.1186/s12875-021-01420-0

16. Grote T, Berens P (2020) On the ethics of algorithmic decision-making in healthcare. J Med Ethics 46:205–211
17. Vincent J-L, Creteur J (2020) Ethical aspects of the COVID-19 crisis: how to deal with an overwhelming shortage of acute beds. Eur Heart J Acute Cardiovasc Care 9(3):248–252. https://doi.org/10.1177/2048872620922788
18. Lavazza A, Garasic MD (2022) What if some patients are more "important" than others? A possible framework for Covid-19 and other emergency care situations. BMC Med Ethics 23:24. https://doi.org/10.1186/s12910-022-00763-2
19. Cloconi C, Economou M, Charalambous A (2022) Burnout, coping and resilience of the cancer care workforce during the SARS-CoV-2: a multinational cross-sectional study. Eur J Oncol Nurs 102204. https://doi.org/10.1016/j.ejon.2022.102204
20. Pappa S, Ntella V, Giannakas T, Giannakoulis VG, Papoutsi E, Katsaounou P (2020) Prevalence of depression, anxiety, and insomnia among healthcare workers during the COVID-19 pandemic: a systematic review and meta-analysis. Brain Behav Immun 88(January):901–907. https://doi.org/10.1016/j.bbi.2020.05.026
21. Barello S, Palamenghi L, Graffigna G (2020) Burnout and somatic symptoms among frontline healthcare professionals at the peak of the Italian COVID-19 pandemic. Psychiatry Res 290. https://doi.org/10.1016/j.psychres.2020.113129
22. Bressi C, Manenti S, Porcellana M, Cevales D, Farina L, Felicioni I, Meloni G, Milone G, Miccolis IR, Pavanetto M, Pescador L, Poddigue M, Scotti L, Zambon A, Corrao G, Lambertenghi-Deliliers G, Invernizzi G (2008) Haemato-oncology and burnout: an Italian survey. Br J Cancer 98(6):1046–1052. https://doi.org/10.1038/sj.bjc.6604270
23. Shaukat N, Ali DM, Razzak J (2020) Physical and mental health impacts of COVID-19 on healthcare workers: a scoping review. Int J Emerg Med 13(1). https://doi.org/10.1186/s12245-020-00299-5
24. Rawlings D, Miller-Lewis L, Tieman J (2022) Impact of the COVID-19 pandemic on funerals: experiences of participants in the 2020 Dying2Learn massive open online course. Omega (United States). https://doi.org/10.1177/00302228221075283
25. Kennedy NR, Steinberg A, Arnold RM, Doshi AA, White DB, DeLair W, Nigra K, Elmer J (2021) Perspectives on telephone and video communication in the intensive care unit during COVID-19. Ann Am Thorac Soc 18(5):838–847. https://doi.org/10.1513/AnnalsATS.202006-729OC
26. Maffoni M, Torlaschi V, Pierobon A, Zanatta F, Grasso R, Bagliani S, Govoni L, Biglieri M, Cerri L, Geraci L, Salvaneschi G, Piaggi G (2021) Video calls during the COVID-19 pandemic: a bridge for patients, families, and respiratory therapists. Fam Syst Health 39(4):650–658. https://doi.org/10.1037/fsh0000661
27. Ehrlich R (2021) Winnicott's idea of the false self: theory as autobiography. J Am Psychoanal Assoc 69(1):75–108. https://doi.org/10.1177/00030651211001461
28. Steiner J (2005) The conflict between mourning and melancholia. Psychoanal Q 74(1):83–104. https://doi.org/10.1002/j.2167-4086.2005.tb00201.x
29. Marcum M, Kurtzweil N, Vollmer C, Schmid L, Vollmer A, Kastl A, Acker K, Gulati S, Grover P, Herzog TJ, Ahmad SA, Sohal D, Wise-Draper TM (2020) COVID-19 pandemic and impact on cancer clinical trials: an academic medical center perspective. Cancer Med 9(17):6141–6146. https://doi.org/10.1002/cam4.3292
30. He Z, Erdengasileng A, Luo X, Xing A, Charness N, Bian J (2021) How the clinical research community responded to the COVID-19 pandemic: an analysis of the COVID-19 clinical studies in ClinicalTrials.gov. JAMIA Open 4(2):ooab032. https://doi.org/10.1093/jamiaopen/ooab032
31. Williams GA, Scarpetti G, Bezzina A, Vincenti K, Grech K, Kowalska-Bobko I, Sowada C, Furman M, Gałązka-Sobotka M, Maier C (2020) Eurohealth 26(2)
32. Juvet TM, Corbaz-Kurth S, Roos P, Benzakour L, Cereghetti S, Moullec G, Suard J-C, Vieux L, Wozniak H, Pralong JA, Weissbrodt R (2021) Adapting to the unexpected: problematic work situations and resilience strategies in healthcare institutions during the COVID-19 pandemic's first wave. Saf Sci 139:105277

Recommended Reading

Cloconi C, Economou M, Charalambous A (2022) Burnout, coping and resilience of the cancer care workforce during the SARS-CoV-2: a multinational cross-sectional study. Eur J Oncol Nurs:102204. https://doi.org/10.1016/j.ejon.2022.102204

Shaukat N, Ali DM, Razzak J (2020) Physical and mental health impacts of COVID-19 on healthcare workers: a scoping review. Int J Emerg Med 13(1):40. https://doi.org/10.1186/s12245-020-00299-5. PMID: 32689925; PMCID: PMC7370263

Open Access This chapter is licensed under the terms of the Creative Commons Attribution 4.0 International License (http://creativecommons.org/licenses/by/4.0/), which permits use, sharing, adaptation, distribution and reproduction in any medium or format, as long as you give appropriate credit to the original author(s) and the source, provide a link to the Creative Commons license and indicate if changes were made.

The images or other third party material in this chapter are included in the chapter's Creative Commons license, unless indicated otherwise in a credit line to the material. If material is not included in the chapter's Creative Commons license and your intended use is not permitted by statutory regulation or exceeds the permitted use, you will need to obtain permission directly from the copyright holder.

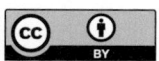

The Effect of the COVID-19 Pandemic on the Charity Sector

7

Dany Bell

Check Your Experience
1. If you work in healthcare, how has the use of virtual support provided by charities over the course of the COVID-19 pandemic supported your patient group?
2. What did your patients, and their families, value and access from charities to support their cancer care?

Introduction

The term charity is used as shorthand to refer to the range of non-profit and social sector organisations referred to in this chapter. Charities were at the sharp end of the COVID-19 crisis [1] which saw the impact on National Health Service (NHS) charities as needing to work harder to support healthcare workers across care settings, and other charities such as domestic abuse hotlines, and cancer charity helplines who experienced spikes in call rates, so charities had to quickly adapt to support the increased need [1].

Charities provide a mix of services such as helplines, volunteer visiting and practical help, walk-in services, bereavement visiting and much more. For many the face-to-face services are a large proportion of their work. Subsequently, as well as seeing increased demand, charities had to shift their face-to-face support services to online with barely any preparation time. Alongside this, thousands of fundraising events were cancelled, and it was clear that charities were in no doubt that the pandemic presented significant long-term challenges to them financially.

Charity organisations' work also supports the health and social care sector which was under severe pressure throughout the pandemic and beyond. Both the charitable and the health and social care sectors were very concerned about the support and

D. Bell (✉)
Macmillan Cancer Support, London, UK
e-mail: DaBell@macmillan.org.uk

© The Authors(s) 2026
M. Foulkes et al. (eds.), *Cancer Care in the Post-COVID World*,
https://doi.org/10.1007/978-3-031-33855-7_7

care of cancer patients from the early days of the COVID-19 pandemic, beyond, into recovery and the 'new normal' of workforce and capacity pressures. These concerns ranged from access and delivery of key diagnostic tests and treatment to the support people required for physical, psychosocial, practical and financial concerns.

Charitable sector work is often preventative as it intervenes early, often reaching communities and individuals that public and government agencies struggle to reach. They campaign and advocate for the most vulnerable in our society, empowering and giving people with lived experience a much-needed voice. It could be advocated that voluntary organisations are the social glue within our society as they are the places where people come together so they can solve shared problems, share passions and interests, and throughout that process, communities are built and strengthened, allowing trust between individuals and organisations to be generated and collaboration and co-production to take place [2].

Another important link between the NHS and charities comes in the form of social prescribing [3], a term used to describe the referral of patients from primary care to a wide range of local non-clinical services for a variety of support. Social prescribing has been formalised in recent years with the introduction of 'link workers'—roles in the primary care team who take on patients from general practitioners, assess their needs and signpost them to services that could help and support them.

A large proportion of the services that link workers engage with are charities that were massively affected by the COVID-19 pandemic, and many lost 70% of their funds due to their fundraising being halted due to the necessary restrictions. Many professionals rely on charities, often referring patients to them for mental and physical health support, bereavement and homelessness. This meant charities had to rapidly reinvent the way they delivered support to maintain a presence and continue to deliver that vital support.

The Charity Commission explored the impact on charities in England and Wales and how they adapted during the pandemic and produced several reports [4]. Finding that some charities were quickly able to move to provide services online demonstrating there was an acceleration of digital transformation within the charitable sector during the COVID-19 pandemic, where progress in this area prior to this had been slow often due to the cost. For others, this was not an option due to the nature of their charitable activity, for example, indoor or outdoor group activity all undertaken face to face which could not continue and, ultimately, left a gap in support and compounded isolation. Essentially, they found that nearly all charities (91%) in England and Wales experienced some negative impact from the COVID-19 pandemic. The consequences spanned service delivery, finances and staffing issues, as well as frustration and uncertainty due to the rapidly changing environment.

The Scottish Charity Regulator (OSCR) [5] also undertook a survey to understand how Scottish charities had adapted during the pandemic. Some charities became involved in running food banks or provided shopping and prescription delivery services; delivered meals to support people who were isolated, vulnerable, or shielding; and others diversified into new types of community support programmes and projects that brought the wider communities together virtually.

The Charities Aid Foundation (CAF) [6, 7] undertook research interviewing a representative sample of the public each month across 2020, with the goal of assisting charities, government and wider society to better understand the United Kingdom's giving landscape and the global impact on charities. CAF is registered in the United Kingdom, America and Canada. They worked with their global alliance partners to conduct extensive research across a range of countries (South Africa, Brazil, Australia, Turkey, India, the United Kingdom, America, Russia). Key findings were:

- A shift of staff to remote working.
- Developed alternative or innovative ways to deliver their support services.
- Found new ways to reach people they support.
- Refocused their charitable activities.
- Developed new collaborations with organisations.
- Used financial support to pay salaries of their staff.
- Invested in new technology.
- Undertook emergency fundraising campaigns.

However, some charities had to stop or reduce their services, and some were viewed as non-essential by their governments [7]. Many charities from all countries received donations of goods from either individuals or corporations during the crisis that they could utilise to support people, for example, a donation of iPads meant these could be distributed to people in need to stay connected. Surprising to many charities was the willingness of volunteers and public support for them, in much the same way they were supporting and championing health and social care, at a difficult time for everyone.

What was perhaps universal was for charities to question their purpose during the COVID-19 pandemic and continue to help in the most practical way possible, whilst making tough decisions about finances and staff. However, many charities rose to the challenge and delivered innovation and formed partnerships that would stand the test of time and continue beyond the pandemic. In the UK partnerships developed between a wide range of charities. These included a collaboration between leading mental health charities, i.e., Mind, Samaritans, Shout and Hospice UK, to create a mental health platform to help those providing frontline support for those affected by the COVID-19 pandemic. At a local level, collaboration across small charities increased, matching charities and businesses together to ensure their communities' needs were being met during the pandemic.

Technology

For many charities their pandemic response allowed them to work more collaboratively and mobilise quickly around common goals, developing new ways of working which were more agile and responsive. Part of this new era was using digital platforms to enable continued delivery of services, and whilst digital transformation has been slow in the third sector [8], it was necessary for them to continue to reach people, fundraise and provide much-needed services which required a digital approach. Some did this by redirecting funds due to inability to continue some services, by collaborating and sharing the cost or finding ways to access funding sources. Training was provided by staff not furloughed working within these collaborations, for example, Macmillan Cancer Support partnered with Wessex Cancer Alliance, Southampton University and 'CanRehab' (providers of evidence-based, specialist training in Cancer and Exercise in the United Kingdom) to develop a virtual rehabilitation model which utilised electronic need assessments which Macmillan trained 'CanRehab' staff to use. Subsequently a National Institute for Healthcare Research (NIHR) bid was successful to scale this up and research the impact and viability of this as a long-term model.

Gilliland (2020) [8] highlighted that 51% of charities in the United Kingdom did not have a digital strategy at the time of the pandemic, and what the COVID-19 pandemic did was shine a light on the fact that people who often need the most support are those who are not digitally mature. This meant that the third sector had to be more strategic in using the right tools to reach their audiences and highlighted the need for digital skills within charities and the communities they support.

The COVID-19 Voluntary Sector Impact Barometer (2021) [9], led by the National Council for Voluntary Organisations (NCVO), Nottingham Trent University and Sheffield Hallam University, highlighted that changes in how technology was being used in the charitable sector led to improvements in digital service accessibility with 45% of 350 charities surveyed having reported improved accessibility, as a result of investing in new technology and ensuring volunteers had the skills to use it, whilst 17% reported reduced accessibility.

Many charities had to invest in technology to enable their staff to work remotely [9]. Whilst others had to use traditional methods to reach audiences, such as implementing a range of telephone services in addition to any helpline support to deliver different kinds of support. For example, Macmillan Cancer Support utilised its volunteers to offer a telephone buddy service for people isolated [10], and Lloyds bank teamed up with charities to ensure those over 70 remained connected which included a dedicated phone line delivered by We Are Digital to provide guidance and remote training to support them with everyday digital activities, after We Are Digital supplied free iPads [11]. They also worked with Mental Health UK and The Silver Line (partner with Age UK) to provide both practical and emotional support to help mitigate the effects of COVID-19 on the nation's mental health.

Due to the higher demand on helplines with the main queries on shielding guidance and cancelled treatments, charities had to explore implementing other methods like text services and chatbots to enable their support staff to have the ability to cope with the increased demand [12–14].

However, there were barriers and challenges highlighted by The Digital Skills report in 2020 [15]:

- Lack of funding was the biggest barrier to getting more from digital for 50% of charities.
- Staff skills came out as the second biggest barrier, with 48% of respondents selecting this.

Overall, one in five charities had poor skills across a range of areas of digital, including user needs, data, analytics, cybersecurity, digital service delivery and digital fundraising.

Therefore, the enforced pivot to digital that many charitable organisations had to make during the pandemic brought new challenges, but also opened opportunities for new ways of working to deliver on their mission. So, it is fair to say that over the last two years, the third sector has gone through a period of intense digital adaptation. The Charity Commission [4] surveyed charity trustees and the public to understand the impact 1 year on. They found that 38% of charities had moved services online. This was as high as 63% for charities with income over £500,000, whereas for charities with income under £10,000, it was only 24%. The Charity Digital Skills report (2022) [16] found that 66% of charities are now delivering all work remotely, and 47% are collaborating and sharing learning with others around their digital experience. Equally, for the first time since 2012, there was a percentage move back in favour of the importance of charities from the public due to their response in exceptional circumstances during COVID [17].

Innovation of Services

Research from the Pro Bono Economics COVID Charity Tracker [18], produced in partnership with Charity Finance Group and the Chartered Institute of Fundraising, showed that there was widespread innovation throughout the charity sector because of the COVID-19 pandemic.

Shifting the Balance [19] highlighted genuine innovations emerged during the pandemic—brand new neighbourhood networks, entirely new funding schemes and original partnerships that connected different kinds of community businesses, voluntary groups and charities. For example, Monmouthshire County Council and the third sector worked together to build a support structure for community groups. This involved training and screening volunteers for safeguarding, sharing information, building neighbourhood networks so that community groups could help each other and providing a single point of contact in the council who could assist groups with any challenges they were experiencing. 'Look after each other' was the single purpose that brought Sheffield's public services and communities together in the first lockdown. The city pulled together and forgot about their job descriptions. Energised by a can-do culture and aided by swift decision-making processes, they used whatever skills and expertise they had to support others however they could. More grants were handed over by public bodies directly to communities for them to develop their own responses and spend on their own priorities.

The scale and urgency of the COVID-19 pandemic crisis made agility and speed non-negotiable for all involved; it was a must. Therefore, usual bureaucracy and processes were scaled back so that swift responses to urgent needs were prioritised. Everyone's incentives shifted toward resolving problems as collaboratively and rapidly as possible.

Charities gathered valuable insight to ensure they could meet the physical and psychological needs of people with cancer, subsequently developing virtual offers to support the physical and emotional well-being of all their audiences—people with cancer, professionals who support them and carers managing non-medical care. These ranged from resources in video format on their websites to partnering with organisations to develop virtual prehabilitation [20] and rehabilitation to support people through treatment and longer-term recovery. Some of these innovations had research partners to gather the evidence that would enable longevity [21]. Whilst the final evidence is being gathered, the intended outcomes for the virtual prehabilitation are optimisation of training package, providing a model for future implementation. Upskilling the workforce to contribute to the care offered throughout the cancer pathway helps provide the holistic support that will benefit people affected by cancer.

Innovative partnerships and the use of digital to ensure people had access to counselling and mental health support virtually were developed due to the impact of the COVID-19 pandemic on mental health [22]. For example, in Northern Ireland, unprecedented expertise with one clear aim—to support mental health and well-being of people—came together by way of the Department for Communities and the Department of Health partnering with 15 leading mental and well-being health charities and the Healthy Living Centre Alliance representing 28 local healthy living centres to focus on promoting mental health and well-being during and after the COVID-19 pandemic [23]. Macmillan Cancer Support partnered with BUPA (a UK provider of private healthcare) to ensure those that needed skilled intervention from trained professionals for mental health could receive this for free [24]. The aim of the service was for people with cancer to be able to access up to six free remote (online or by phone) counselling sessions, tailored to meet the specific needs of each individual and designed to help them understand, manage and overcome difficult feelings. There was internal training required by the helpline staff to be able to triage people with psychological needs requiring psychological intervention. There was a worry about huge demand and cost, but in fact, it was a success and subsequently changed to a Macmillan service that professionals could signpost to, rather than only accessible via the Macmillan helpline.

Whilst some charities scaled down or closed services, some like SignHealth [25] (a charity promoting good health and well-being for deaf people) expanded their services to meet the need by:

- Translating over 150 government briefings, 6 shielding letters and other documents to ensure people had COVID-19 information in Brail and sign language (BSL).
- Launching BSL Health, ensuring deaf people had free remote access to all health settings nationwide facilitating 42,000 calls through the pandemic.
- Working with UK COVID 'Test and Trace' and test centres to ensure accessibility for deaf people.
- Producing the 'About Me' well-being plan for deaf people isolating.

There was also innovation at the local level, as when the COVID-19 pandemic hit, many community charity organisations providing much-needed local support had to shut down [26]. So, these organisations big and small had to reassess the needs within their communities and how they could support people. The imagination and resourcefulness at the local level to create innovation during lockdowns demonstrated the creativity and resilience of the charitable sector with armies of volunteers supporting those most at risk by way of projects such as [26]:

- 'Zoom cafes' replacing luncheon clubs
- 'Dial a story'—programme that enables children and adults to dial their local library from any telephone and listen to taped stories
- Doorstep fitness.
- App-based food vouchers.

From the outset of the COVID-19 pandemic, charities showed great strength in adapting to the challenges the pandemic presented, particularly working together as they transferred service delivery online [9].

Resilience

Working in the voluntary sector can be enormously demanding, requiring resilience for many reasons, for example, the work can be emotional and distressing. However, those working in the sector feel a huge privilege to work with people and communities, witnessing the passion, dedication and skills within their charity teams and other charitable organisations. Equally supporting people who are struggling, with stretched resources, can take its toll on the staff, volunteers and leaders of charities, so ensuring adequate access to support is vital, and many have their own well-being offer for staff.

The COVID-19 pandemic hit charities and the people they work with particularly hard. Charities sought to continue and expand services and support for communities in real need. For these user-led organisations, this tension was particularly intense, as many were experiencing the same needs for support as their beneficiaries.

Ensuring staff well-being was a priority for charities, including support for staff furloughed, and those whose own illness or long-term condition placed them at risk.

Many teams found ways to undertake joint activity virtually, like team quizzes or virtual coffee breaks. For some it was not ideal working remotely as sometimes people did not have the right space, which required appropriate action and flexibility in working arrangements for people with no space for a desk often using what was available. These staff were given priority to return to the office when restrictions permitted as many charities had to reduce office space to save money at the height of the pandemic and review access to the office as a result when restrictions were relaxed more. Despite the difficulties with the right support, staff remained resilient and passionate about the purpose of their organisation and continued to be creative and innovative.

The 2022 UK Charitable Giving Research report [27] highlighted that adaptability, innovation and collaboration in the face of crisis were central to the resilience of UK charities and volunteers, despite unclear guidance and support. The survey shows how across the period surveyed UK charities reported concern about their finances; saw rising demand for their services; navigated falls in income, staffing and volunteer numbers; and adapted to a world moving online to successfully support their audiences.

It is fair to say that the COVID-19 pandemic's effect on cancer patients was, and remains, a key concern to the cancer charity and health communities, and charities strived hard against challenges to continue to support people throughout the pandemic. In its second COVID-19-era survey, CAF America [7] polled 880 organisations worldwide to learn how the coronavirus global pandemic continued to impact their work. Despite nearly all charities being negatively affected by the pandemic, they found that many continued to successfully continue their operations, due to three overall determining factors: access to technology and the ability to move operations online; their team's commitment, adaptability and creativity; and access to continued funding.

Roberta Fusco, Director of Policy and Communications at Charity Finance Group [18], highlighted 'charities and social change organisations have shown huge amounts of resilience, adaptability and decisive action through 2020. Charities have stepped up to deliver at pace and have pulled all the levers at their disposal'.

The Kreston Charities Survey 2021 [25] highlighted that:

- More than 95% of charities questioned were financially resilient during the pandemic.
- Almost 80% were happy with current reserve levels.
- 65% expected income to increase.
- 97% believed they would survive the next 12 months.
- 70% expected a further increase in demand for their services.
- 53% had accessed the coronavirus job retention scheme.
- 18% had access to the coronavirus community support fund.
- Over 70% were envisaging a blended mix of face-to-face and online activity.

It also highlighted that the changing work practices implemented during the pandemic were expected to remain, including flexible working, more digital and online services and mental health and well-being support for employees. These positive findings, particularly the innovations nearly all felt would survive the next 12 months, demonstrate how resilient the sector was in coping with the challenges of the COVID-19 pandemic, in particular the financial challenges.

Equally charities collaborated effectively with each other and with other business organisations, proving to be extremely flexible in their response to the pandemic and all its challenges. The benefits of successful collaboration included greater efficiency and use of resources, improved services and a stronger voice and influence.

The resilience of charities through the pandemic may be the result of their willingness and ability to take steps to address the immediate challenges facing them with their actions having had a significant impact on the way charities now deliver services to their beneficiaries.

Fundraising

Against the backdrop of the global pandemic and associated recession, any assessment of the impact on the income of charities needed to consider three key questions [4]:

1. Where charity funding comes from?
2. What factors drive that income?
3. What is likely to happen to those driving factors over the course of the post-pandemic recession and recovery?

Before the COVID-19 pandemic, charity funding came from the public via donations, legacies and shops/charity goods sold online. The government accounted for a further 29% of the charity total, investment returns added another 8%, and the remainder was drawn from foundations, corporations and the National Lottery [4].

The majority (**60%**) saw a loss of income, and a third (**32%**) said they experienced a shortage of volunteers [4]. Given these findings, it is perhaps surprising that a significant number of charities have not folded since the start of the pandemic. Overall, the number of charities closing did not vary significantly across 2020 and 2021, with 97 charities out of 170,000 on the Charity Commission register folding in 2020 and similar in 2021 [4].

In the United Kingdom, the Charity Commission [4] highlighted changes charities made in the face of financial challenges, which varied across the sector. According to their research:

- Around half of charities with income over £500,000 used furlough or emergency government support, but smaller charities were much less likely to have done so due to uncertainty of being able to employ staff beyond the pandemic [26].
- Smaller charities were more likely to have stopped services—25% of charities with an income under £10,000 stopped all services, compared to 3% of charities over £500,000.

The Charity Commission also held round tables to hear some of the stories behind these numbers. These included measures like:

- Taking different approaches to fundraising.
- Developing new business and revenue models.
- Trustee boards working in new ways to respond to financial and governance challenges.

Global Alliance CAF partner report [7] highlighted that 60% of non-governmental organisations (NGOs) recorded a decrease in donations between March and April 2020, and it is fair to say this was the picture across the board in many countries throughout 2020 with many charities predicting 30–50% loss in income for that financial year.

In an ever-changing environment, charities needed to be flexible but so did their funders. As a response to the pandemic, the report shows that charities saw many funders pivot to provide emergency support and adopt a more flexible approach. By allowing grants to be repurposed or requirements relaxed, organisations were able to respond to crises that they faced. However, this tended to benefit organisations with already strong networks.

Recovery

In 2021 Wood [1] explored how charities, with the support of the government and grant funders, could come back stronger from the trials of the COVID-19 pandemic to become more resilient and capable of fulfilling the crucial role they play during recovery. This would be achieved through learning lessons around digital delivery and fundraising, remote working and diversifying fundraising strategies.

CAF researched the charity landscape for 2022 [27] from the perspective of 547 UK charity leaders. Of those, 58% said that generating income and finding financial stability were among their top three challenges for the year ahead. A similar percentage (59%) are concerned that people will not donate to their cause because of the cost-of-living crisis. With less disposable income and food and fuel prices rising, charities cannot rely on the monetary support of their communities. These concerns are warranted as one in seven people said they intend to reduce their charity donations this year.

The Charity Commission [4] published a report on the impact of the COVID-19 pandemic on charities showing that 60% had experienced a loss of income. CAF's research in 2022 [26] suggests that this loss of income is likely to continue.

The National Council for Voluntary Organisations (NCVO) published a report in March 2022 [25], as they had tracked the pandemic's impact on voluntary, community and social organisations throughout 2020 and 2021. It found that nearly half of the organisations surveyed had reverted to using cash reserves to continue operating during the pandemic and almost two-thirds anticipated future financial difficulties.

Overall, the impact of the pandemic on the charitable sector's services is highly mixed. Whilst the headline picture is one of significantly increased demands across the board, the reality is a little more nuanced. Some charities have experienced a significant drop in demand for some or all services they deliver and have had to respond accordingly.

The voluntary sector played a vital role in responding to the challenges of the pandemic. The sector's agility in responding to differing needs was impressive, and this was despite some of the difficulties the sector was already facing pre-pandemic.

The long-term outlook for the third sector has remained uncertain, particularly for smaller organisations that rely on public fundraising for their income. Despite reduced income and capacity to provide services, charity organisations faced higher than ever demands. In the short term, had to modify how services were delivered, including moving some activities online to continue supporting service users, carers and the wider health system. The increased use of technology has been beneficial for the sector as it has allowed wider reach and enabled a hybrid offer to continue as people returned to work and normal life, enabling people to choose how they access support.

Increased use of digital services was not without its challenges, however, and organisations needed to ensure their online provision was and remains accessible and suitable for the needs of their service users [9]. Further developing volunteer capacity remains an important opportunity for the sector to build a sustainable workforce, equipped to deliver services. Roles for volunteers during Covid included acting as local community champions and working alongside paid staff in public sector organisations, engaging and understanding the lived experience through Covid and beyond. Reforming services that addressed health inequalities and improved well-being for the people who were the worst affected by the pandemic is a continued priority.

Nine lessons learned by charities from COVID-19 [9]:

1. Embedding flexible funding practices beyond the pandemic.
2. Creating more longer-term funding opportunities.
3. Increasing charity collaboration and support for the charity ecosystem.
4. Rethinking the roles of communities and volunteering.
5. Improving the diversity of charity leaders and trustees.
6. Increasing inclusion and well-being within charities.
7. Encouraging flexible working and volunteering.
8. Addressing digital exclusion and upskilling the charity workforce.
9. Funding and support to build digital resilience in charities.

Test Your Learning
1. Has the adoption of virtual support that commenced during the COVID-19 pandemic and continued by cancer charities impacted how you support your patients?
2. What evidence is required to ensure adoption of virtual support services by charities remains meaningful to patients?

References

1. Wood C (2021) The impact of the COVID-19 pandemic on the charitable sector and its prospects for recovery' DEMOS, 15 Whitehall, London, SW1A 2DD
2. National Lottery (2018) Putting good ingredients in the mix – lessons and opportunities for place-based working and funding. Big Lottery Fund, 2018 Version 1. Published in August 2018. https://www.tnlcommunityfund.org.uk/media/documents/BLF_KL18-11-Place-Based-Funding.pdf. Last accessed June 2023
3. Mahase E (2020) Covid-19: charity cuts could put the NHS under even more pressure. BMJ https://doi.org/10.1136/bmj.m3261. Last accessed June 2023
4. Charity Commission (2021) Charity Commission COVID-19 Survey 2021. https://www.gov.uk/government/publications/charity-commission-covid-19-survey-2021. Last accessed July 2023
5. OSCR (2020) How charities adapted to the pandemic. https://www.oscr.org.uk/media/4231/062021-how-charities-adapted-to-the-pandemic.pdf. Last accessed July 2023
6. Charities Aid Foundation (2020) UK giving and COVID-19: a special report. https://www.cafonline.org/about-us/publications/2020-publications/uk-giving-2020. Last accessed July 2023
7. Charities Aid Foundation (2020) COVID-19: lessons in disaster philanthropy: the voice of charities facing COVID-19', vol. 1–8. https://www.cafamerica.org/covid19reports/. Last accessed July 2023
8. Gilliland N (2020) How digital priorities have changed for charities since Covid-19' eConsultancy report. https://econsultancy.com/how-digital-priorities-have-changed-for-charities-since-covid-19/. Last accessed July 2023
9. Nottingham Trent University (2022) Respond, recover, reset: the voluntary sector and COVID-19. http://cpwop.org.uk/what-we-do/projects-and-publications/covid-19-vcse-organisation-responses. Last accessed July 2023
10. Howell M (2020) 'Sometimes you really need a hug': how Macmillan's telephone buddies help isolated cancer patients. Daily Telegraph, December 12th, 2020. https://www.telegraph.co.uk/christmas/2020/12/12/sometimes-really-need-hug-macmillans-telephone-buddies-help/. Last accessed July 2023
11. Lloyds Bank (2020) Press release – Lloyds Banking Group teams up with we are digital, the silver line and mental health UK to offer practical and emotional support for the most vulnerable in society during the coronavirus crisis. https://www.lloydsbankinggroup.com/assets/pdfs/media/press-releases/2020-press-releases/lloyds-banking-group/20200414-societal-response-corporate-media-release-final.pdf. Last accessed July 2023
12. World Health Organisation (2022) Chatbots against COVID-19: using chatbots to answer questions on COVID-19 in the user's language. https://www.who.int/news-room/feature-stories/detail/scicom-compilation-chatbot. Last accessed July 2023
13. Miller K (2020) How Chatbots are helping with Covid-19'@very well health. https://www.verywellhealth.com/how-chatbots-can-help-with-covid-19-5070338. Last accessed July 2023
14. News and Star, The Cumberland News (2020) Arthritis charity launches Chatbot to offer Covid-19. https://www.newsandstar.co.uk/news/national/18378228.arthritis-charity-launches-chatbot-offer-covid-19-advice/. Last accessed July 2023
15. Amar Z (2020) Charity digital skills report 2020. https://www.skillsplatform.org/uploads/charity_digital_skills_report_2020.pdf. Last accessed July 2023
16. Amar Z (2022) Charity digital skills report 2022. https://charitydigitalskills.co.uk/download-the-charity-digital-skills-report/. Last accessed July 2023
17. The Charity Commission (2021) Trust in charities post COVID. https://www.gov.uk/government/publications/public-trust-in-charities-and-trustees-experience-of-their-role/public-trust-in-charities-2021-web-version. Last accessed July 2023

18. Pro Bono Economics (2021) The charity sector through COVID – in partnership with charity finance group and the chartered institute of fundraising. https://ciof.org.uk/events-and-training/resources/the-charity-sector-through-covid. Last accessed July 2023
19. Kaye S, Morgan C (2021) Shifting the balance: local adaptation, innovation and collaboration during the pandemic and beyond. https://www.newlocal.org.uk/wp-content/uploads/2021/01/Shifting-the-Balance.pdf. Last accessed July 2023
20. Wessex Cancer Alliance (2023) SafeFit. https://wessexcanceralliance.nhs.uk/safefit/. Last accessed July 2023
21. Grimmett C et al (2021) SafeFit trial: virtual clinics to deliver a multimodal intervention to improve psychological and physical wellbeing in people with cancer. Protocol of a Covid-19 targeted non-randomised phase III trial. BMJ Open 11(8)
22. Xiong J et al (2020) Impact of COVID-19 pandemic on mental health in the general population: a systematic review. J Affect Disord 277:55–64
23. The Department for Communities Northern Ireland (2021) Government and charities join forces to support mental wellbeing. https://www.communities-ni.gov.uk/news/government-and-charities-join-forces-support-mental-wellbeing. Last accessed July 2023
24. Macmillan Cancer Support and BUPA (2021) Free counselling service. https://www.macmillan.org.uk/cancer-information-and-support/get-help/emotional-help/bupa-counselling-and-emotional-well-being-support. Last accessed July 2023
25. Owen C (2021) Kreston global charities report. Kreston-Charities-Report-August-2021.pdf. Last accessed July 2023
26. Charities Aid Foundation (2022) UK giving report 2022. https://www.cafonline.org/docs/default-source/about-us-research/uk_giving_2022.pdf. Last accessed July 2023
27. Lloyds Bank Foundation (2020) Small charities responding to COVID-19 winter update. https://www.lloydsbankfoundation.org.uk/influencing/research/charities-responding-to-covid-winter-update. Last accessed July 2023

Recommended Reading

Comas-Herrera A, Fernandez JL, Hancock R, Hatton C, Knapp M, McDaid D, Malley J, Wistow G, Wittenberg R (2020) COVID-19: implications for the support of people with social care needs in England. J Aging Soc Policy 32(4, 5). https://doi.org/10.1080/08959420.2020.1759759

Kamal MM (2020) The triple-edged sword of COVID-19: understanding the use of digital technologies and the impact of productive, disruptive, and destructive nature of the Pandemic C. Inf Syst Manag 37(4):310–317. https://doi.org/10.1080/10580530.2020.1820634

Kings Fund (2021) Making an impact: small and medium sized voluntary organisations' responses to the COVID-19 pandemic. https://www.kingsfund.org.uk/blog/2021/01/small-medium-voluntary-sector-organisations-responses-covid-19

Madden M, Walton R, Roche M (2020) Going viral. COVID-19: how have charities responded to the first phase of the crisis? nfpSynergy, London

Marmot M, Allen J, Goldblatt P, Herd E, Morrison J (2020) Build back fairer: the COVID-19 Marmot review. The Health Foundation, Institute of Health Equity, London

Open Access This chapter is licensed under the terms of the Creative Commons Attribution 4.0 International License (http://creativecommons.org/licenses/by/4.0/), which permits use, sharing, adaptation, distribution and reproduction in any medium or format, as long as you give appropriate credit to the original author(s) and the source, provide a link to the Creative Commons license and indicate if changes were made.

The images or other third party material in this chapter are included in the chapter's Creative Commons license, unless indicated otherwise in a credit line to the material. If material is not included in the chapter's Creative Commons license and your intended use is not permitted by statutory regulation or exceeds the permitted use, you will need to obtain permission directly from the copyright holder.

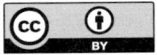

Impact on Cancer Education COVID-19

Karen Campbell

Check Your Experience
1. How has the increased use of technology within your formal and informal cancer courses changed over the course of the COVID-19 pandemic?
2. What are the benefits and challenges reported for maintaining the education mediums utilised in the COVID-19 pandemic?
3. Is there anything that we should maintain in our education courses post-pandemic?

Introduction

Healthcare professional education is at the core of effective, efficient and evidenced delivery of cancer care across Europe. During the pandemic, like most other clinical services, the cessation of in-person activity required a response and shift of education to virtual classrooms or online platforms globally [1]. Like clinical practice, health service education providers, higher education institutions (HEI), cancer and nursing society charities and other established company education providers had to mobilise quickly. The focus was on replacing existing face-to-face provision including clinical skills, whilst embracing training of new skills to support the 'virtual' nature of clinical practice and virtual education. Each sector of education provision had its own priority. These priorities will be discussed further in the chapter and conclude with lessons learnt and the opportunities that could be maintained post-COVID-19 pandemic.

K. Campbell (✉)
School of Health and Social Care, Edinburgh Napier University, Edinburgh, UK
e-mail: K.campbell@napier.ac.uk

© The Author(s) 2026
M. Foulkes et al. (eds.), *Cancer Care in the Post-COVID World*,
https://doi.org/10.1007/978-3-031-33855-7_8

Response to Educating Cancer Healthcare Professionals the Higher Education Institutions (HEI) Perspective

During the COVID-19 pandemic, cancer healthcare workforces were responding by setting up new virtual services or being redeployed to other clinical areas. The shift in workforce meant that many heath care professionals had to halt their personal development pathways and replace with either new skill sets or new qualifications.

The ability of post-graduate students to continue their studies varied and the response of the HEI would have been variable and dependent on their geographical regions and relationships with their NHS providers. Numerous HEIs were shutting down with a COVID emergency response, where most post-graduate courses were given special dispensation to be suspended. Other institutions may have dealt with requests for special education outputs and training to support the virtual clinical world. This would have led to negative consequences for some and opportunities for other healthcare professionals. Initially the HEI may have halted their postgraduate provision, but at the same time, most HEIs were transitioning their face-to-face and residential courses into online format for both post and undergraduate students.

The Response for Online Provision

Online provision is not a new concept in cancer education [2]. However, the majority of HEI provisions that was delivered face to face now had to be delivered online. This response, in the main, was not what is considered the 'gold standard' of online and e-learning. The initial response was to replicate a known way of teaching through virtual learning environments. How much this was underpinned by pedagogical online learning theory depended on the institutional knowledge, experience and the infrastructure available to the HEI staff [3]. Therefore, through the pandemic, there may have been an iterative approach to the design and development and delivery of education, as the HEI staff were taught key principles of how to create engagement, motivation and socialisation for effective education within the online environment [4].

Moving towards living post-COVID, this has created a new language in academic education in general. Consider that we have moved away from the terminology of face-to-face education to in-person. This has emerged as we can have effective face-to-face conversations online. Therefore, a new concept had to be devised to express the environment in which face-to-face teaching can be achieved. As we emerge from COVID so will the language change in respect to the type of education provision. HEIs are now talking about *blended by design* to distinguish from the immediate response to the development of online education. *Flipped classroom* activity (a pre-lecture, then tutorial instead of the didactic lecture style) has become more popular from a student perspective, enabling flexibility [5]. As the technology infrastructure improves, *hybrid* options in education are increasing with some attending in-person and others remotely simultaneously. Similarities in language changes are mirrored in the conference setting, which will be discussed later in this chapter.

Even though the online infrastructure has provided a basis on which HEIs could mobilise quickly, this chapter cannot be written without considering how this change in provision impacts the institution, staff and student personal circumstances. Mohammad and Khalaf [6] state in their literature review that e-learning has afforded more time to absorb the content than traditional teaching without impacting student communication. E-learning enables repeat watching before in-person tutorial discussion or online discussion board activities. In turn Gillet et al. [7] show how the online virtual fellowship initiative can facilitate critical thinking and interpersonal skills.

Carolan et al. [3] rightly point out that how we move forward will have consequences for the individual, wider society and the planet. Online provision of education can be seen as cost-saving, within the university, but now especially for students who are having to make financial decisions during the emerging economic crisis across Europe. In addition, online education opens a more sustainable global networking capability for our future students, without creating carbon dioxide emissions. Lyapichev et al. [8] question if their pathology fellowships are the future of education or a present reality and conclude that they will continue to provide fellowship opportunities not only to their staff but also, due to a high demand, globally.

Online education cannot be done well without considering the negative aspects of this type of education which included social isolation and the inability to access it due to financial constraints that potentially creates a greater divide between the rich and poor in terms of the acquisition of knowledge. This reinforces that pedagogical principles should underpin education; however, a wider acknowledgement of inequity of access also needs to be addressed post COVID-19 pandemic.

The Response for Clinical Placements

The major priority of the HEI during the pandemic was the future cancer healthcare professional workforce and preparing them for qualification with a confident clinical skill set. The immediate response to the pandemic was to stop all clinical practice placements, then evolving to final year nursing students being deployed and paid to support clinical areas [9]. As the pandemic became more predictable, clinical placements recommenced but with increasing interest in carrying these out in a more simulated or virtual environment. To this end 'virtual placements' have been trialled and shown to be effective in education delivery: peer-enhanced e-placements (PEEP model) in occupational therapy courses [10], social work [11], newly qualified oncology nurses [7] and student nursing [12].

These innovations propelled the HEIs into thinking differently about the delivery of clinical skills within the undergraduate healthcare professional programmes. COVID-19 supported through necessity innovations which would have taken the securing of funding and randomised controlled trials to convince a change of practice. However, post pandemic, a further driver will be the capacity requirements for clinical areas as the necessity to train healthcare professional students increases [10]. Therefore, the practice of 'virtual' placements is here to stay.

Cancer education, across Europe, within undergraduate programmes is reported as variable. To provide cancer 'virtual' placements would ensure that students finish their programmes having experienced either cancer content or clinical placements. Evidence of the success of 'virtual' placements is beginning to emerge within cancer conference programmes and hopefully will soon be in publication for us to be able to review and adopt Europe-wide.

Response of NHS Education Services

Like the HEIs, the NHS education providers had a similar response, ceasing face-to-face provision and turning to online platforms for mandatory and non-mandatory education. Holdsworth et al. [13] provide an example of how webinars supported the implementation of video consultations at pace and scale within allied healthcare professionals. This was built around the 12-week scale-up of the NHS 'Near Me' Video conferencing platform across primary and secondary care in Scotland. Utilising a survey approach, the education team gathered pre- and post-knowledge and confidence scores immediately and after the webinars. They also issued surveys at 4 and 8 weeks to establish the impact on clinical practice. Levels of understanding, knowledge and confidence were found to be statistically significant ($p < 0.001$) with 75.5% of the attendees using the video conferencing on the 8-week follow-up, with allied healthcare professionals contributing to 17% of all the national activity by June 2020. Holdsworth et al. [13] also state that this implementation allowed the immediate upskilling of a diverse and dispersed workforce, enabling safe remote working to be expanded at pace and scale whilst also providing unique impact data on the use of webinars to educate across a wide geographical area.

Response from the Cancer Charity and Nursing Society Community

The pattern of response to the COVID-19 pandemic across cancer charities and nursing societies integrated elements of education provision, but their immediate priorities were to ensure that healthcare professionals had the most updated information to deliver appropriate care. Websites and newsletters became the portal for national guidance to reach thousands of nurses each week. One example of success was a collaboration between Macmillan Cancer Support and UK Oncology Nursing Society (UKONS) issuing a weekly 'breaking news' which saw the membership of UKONS double during the pandemic to access information. The website portals allowed a measurement of the topics of interest to the oncology nursing community including palliative care, care of the dying, bereavement, current treatment options and communication skills for virtual consultations. During subsequent waves of the pandemic, the priority became health and well-being of the workforce.

An immediate response was seen within Macmillan Cancer Support, transforming their existing face-to-face provision and delivering through webinars, virtual classrooms and e-learning platforms. They also developed and designed education provision to mirror the website topics of interest. By delivering 'virtually', Macmillan Cancer Support uncovered benefits of delivering in this format including mixed audience from across the United Kingdom, a significant increase in delegate numbers, cost-savings due to no travelling and venue expenses saved. Other smaller cancer charity organisations delivered webinars to their nursing communities and provided a safe place to discuss the challenges in delivering care during COVID. Macmillan Cancer Support in collaboration with Health Education England (HEE) developed an online course on how to deliver Prehabilitation for Cancer patients (PROSPeR). Again, the response of the charities was dependent upon the existing infrastructure and collaborations affording the ability to respond.

Response Within the Conference Arena

The dissemination of research and best practice is vital in oncology, and one of the major means of bringing this about has been attending, and presenting at, conferences. There has been a network of large oncology conferences across the United Kingdom and Europe for many years, and these occur typically in large cities with good transport links. These can either be of general interest with sessions focused on tumour sites or aspects of care or smaller site-specific conferences (such as in lung or breast cancer). These are largely medically driven events, but are often accompanied by sessions, or even whole programmes, which are of interest to oncology nurses or other members of the healthcare team. Conferences are typically funded via sponsorship by pharmaceutical companies or other companies involved in health care. A good example of this type of conference is the annual European Society for Medical Oncology (ESMO) conference which is run concurrently with the annual European Oncology Nursing Society (EONS) meeting. This provides a huge hub for oncologists, oncology nurses and sponsors to gather, network and share the latest research in the form of oral presentations or posters. It is one of the largest oncology conferences in the world with an attendance of around 25,000. Each country also has a network of smaller oncology conferences with some site specialism and some specialised by occupation. This system of in-person conferences was, in effect, completely dismantled by the pandemic with virtually all events cancelled in both 2020 and 2021. In place of these conferences, there arose a series of virtual events with either pre-recorded or live presentations and with attendees 'logging on' to experience these.

Despite the urgent manner in which these events were established, it quickly became apparent that a new model had emerged for delivering conferencing. This new type of oncology conference is certainly friendlier to the environment as they require no travel. There is no travelling time and hence no travelling budget; the sessions could be accessed from the clinical environments in which attendees worked and could be fitted around their other responsibilities. Could it be that the model of face-to-face conference is no longer relevant in the post-pandemic era? As some traditional conferences return in 2022, this largely remains to be seen, but Dr. David Oliver writing eloquently in the *British Medical Journal* discusses the pros and cons of physically attending large conferences and in the end writes a persuasive piece about their benefits [14]. In the online version, the possibilities for networking are very much reduced, the ability to discuss posters and presentations with the people who produce them is also reduced, and attending online, he argues, is a much less enriching experience than attending in person. The online conference may actually be a less effective way of sharing research and best practice. In the final analysis, it might be that the final arbiter of whether online conferences remain in place over traditional conference formats is the degree to which they can be sponsored by large pharmaceutical companies and other healthcare industries.

Despite the, now ubiquitous, nature of online conferencing, there is little comparative work to suggest how effective the format might be. In work that predates the pandemic, Maria Jose Sa and her fellow researchers [15] conducted a literature review and found that the virtual format may enhance academic participation, reducing some inequalities resulting from factors such as gender, race/ethnicity or social class but indicated that a hybrid approach combining both in-person and virtual elements might fulfil the needs of a majority of stakeholders. The hybrid approach to conferencing is a very new one, and the methodologies are in their infancy. Outside of oncology, Puccinelli et al. [16] considered the challenges and comparative advantages and disadvantages of running hybrid conferences. The conclusions reached were that hybrid conferences offered a higher level of flexibility to participants as online only cannot replace either the direct interactions present in an in-person event. They also recognised, however, that hybrid conferences are currently more expensive to run.

Future Provision

As we emerge from the last 2 years of responding to the needs of the workforce and patients, there is a chance to adopt innovations that have provided an evidence base for a continuation in practice regardless of the pandemic. Before the chapter moves forward to the future of cancer education, it may help to reposition ourselves with the context prior to the COVID-10 pandemic.

Campbell et al. [2], in their systematic review, detail that online education for cancer nursing had a limited evidence base globally. There was a high number of initiatives measuring satisfaction, fewer used self-reported knowledge and confidence levels with a handful measuring impact on patient care. In addition, Dean [16] reported that even if the education was available and compulsory, cancer nurses were doing the education in their own time, even to fulfil service and their NMC validation [17]. Many were using their annual leave and own money to support the continuous development needs. The 2019 Macmillan Cancer Support report *Voices from the Frontline* [18] pointed towards a lack of protected time, funding and locally available course. Dean [19] further supports a lack of robust evaluation evidence to demonstrate the impact that education is improving practice. In addition, this chapter has had to draw upon general healthcare publication with only Gillet et al. [7] focusing upon the qualified oncology fellowship.

So, with a lack of evidence base for practice, if we fast forward to the post-COVID world, Potter and Taylor [20] in a recent editorial identify the necessity to have an immediate recovery plan to support the already stretched cancer workforce [21, 22]. No action risks a shortage of cancer nurses and allied health professional (AHP) workforce without the knowledge, skills and capabilities to deliver the care. As part of this recovery response, an ambitious multi-partnership programme, Aspirant Cancer Career and Education Development (ACCEND), is proposed to address the significant challenges and issues that have faced cancer nursing and allied health professional (AHP) workforce for many years, which have been accelerated by the COVID-19 pandemic. The purpose of ACCEND is to provide guidance and direction about the knowledge and capabilities required by nurses and AHPs who care for people affected by cancer in generalist and specialist services in the United Kingdom. Encouragingly this programme of work has an evaluation process embedded into all workstreams and implementation of the education outputs over the coming years facilitating a robust evidence base on different modes of education delivery.

Summary

During the time of the pandemic, an immediate response was required to provide remote education through virtual learning platforms and augmented reality. There has been a wealth of sharing of practice; however, this does not always translate to academic journals in a timely manner. This means that this chapter has limited robust evaluation or research data to synthesise in the discussion. Every education institution had its own immediate education priority, with a developmental approach during different waves of the pandemic. This ranged from information giving for practice to the development of new clinical skills to the health and well-being of the staff. Pre-COVID-19 pandemic, there was an indication that cancer education was already in jeopardy. With a stretched workforce and an increasing cancer population to be cared, a programme of work has been devised to address the educational workforce needs.

Test Your Learning
1. What are the positive impacts of remote learning for cancer education during the COVID-19 pandemic?
2. What evidence do you believe should be gathered to assess education delivered during the pandemic to make appropriate pedagogically informed choices in cancer education?

Recommended Reading

- Aspirant Cancer Career and Education Development programme (ACCEND) https://www.hee.nhs.uk/our-work/cancer-diagnostics/accend. Last Accessed September 2022
- Drury A, Sulosaari V, Sharp L, Ullgren H, de Munter J, Oldenmenger W (2023) The future of cancer nursing in Europe: addressing professional issues in education, research, policy and practice. Eur J Oncol Nurs 63:102271. https://doi.org/10.1016/j.ejon.2023.102271
- McInally W, Taylor V, Diez de Los Rios C, Sulosaari V, Dowling M, Trigoso E, Rodrigues Gomes SM, Cesario Dias Ycn AR, Piskorjanac S, Tanay MA, Hálfdánardóttir H (2023) Innovations in cancer nursing education across Europe. Eur J Oncol Nurs 63:102305. https://doi.org/10.1016/j.ejon.2023.102305
- PRosPer – Cancer Prehabilitation and Rehabilitation Programme https://www.e-lfh.org.uk/programmes/prosper/. Last Accessed September 2022
- Rangachari D, Im A, and Brondfield S (2022) moving from theory to practice in oncology education when virtual is your reality American society of clinical oncology educational book, vol 42, pp. 864–873

References

1. Naciri A, Radid M, Kharbach A, Chemsi G (2021) E-learning in health professions education during the COVID-19 pandemic: a systematic review. J Educ Eval Health Prof 18:27. https://doi.org/10.3352/jeehp.2021.18.27
2. Campbell K, Taylor V, Douglas S (2019) Effectiveness of online cancer education for nurses and allied health professionals; a systematic review using Kirkpatrick evaluation framework. J Cancer Educ 34(2):339–356. https://doi.org/10.1007/s13187-017-1308-2
3. Carolan C, Davies CL, Crookes P, McGhee S, Roxburgh M (2020) COVID 19: disruptive impacts and transformative opportunities in undergraduate nurse education. Nurse Educ Pract 46:102807. https://doi.org/10.1016/j.nepr.2020.102807
4. Regmi K, Jones L (2020) A systematic review of the factors – enablers and barriers – affecting e-learning in health sciences education. BMC Med Educ 20:91. https://doi.org/10.1186/s12909-020-02007-6
5. Kim TH, Kim JS, Yoon HI et al (2021) Medical student education through flipped learning and virtual rotations in radiation oncology during the COVID-19 pandemic: a cross sectional research. Radiat Oncol 16:204. https://doi.org/10.1186/s13014-021-01927-x
6. AlOsta MR, Khalaf IA (2021) Nursing students perception of E-learning during COVID-19 pandemic; a literature review. Medico Legal Update 21(4):269–277. https://doi.org/10.37506/mlu.v21i4.3141
7. Gillett C, Mason S, Fleming L, Mayer DK, Bryant AL (2022) An academic–practice partnership during COVID-19 pandemic: transitioning from a clinical to virtual fellowship. J Clin Nurs 31:347–352. https://doi.org/10.1111/jocn.15817
8. Lyapichev KA, Loghavi S, El Hussein S, Al-Maghrabi H, Xu J, Konoplev S, Medeiros LJ, Khoury JD (2021) Future of education or present reality?: MD Anderson Cancer Center Hematopathology virtual educational platform during the coronavirus disease 2019 (COVID-19) pandemic. Arch Pathol Lab Med 145(11):1350–1354. https://doi.org/10.5858/arpa.2021-0195-SA
9. Swift A et al (2020) COVID-19 and student nurses: a view from England. J Clin Nurs 2020:1–4

10. Taylor L (2020) Clinical placements: online options for learning during COVID-19 and beyond. Available at https://rcni.com/nursing-standard/students/nursing-studies/clinical-placements-online-options-learning-during-covid-19-and-beyond-169581. Last Accessed September 2022
11. Mitchell B, Sarfati D, Stewart M (2022) COVID-19 and beyond: a prototype for remote/virtual social work field placement. Clin Soc Work J 50:3–10. https://doi.org/10.1007/s10615-021-00788-x
12. Walker J (2020) Virtual clinical placement: when practice-based learning goes online available at https://rcni.com/nursing-standard/students/clinical-placements/virtual-clinical-placement-when-practice-based-learning-goes-online-168486. Last Accessed September 2022
13. Holdsworth L, Provan D, Nash G, Beswick M, Curran C, Colhart I, Hunter A (2021) Can webinars support the implementation of video consultations at pace and scale within the allied health professions? Br J Healthc Manag 27(2):1–9
14. Oliver D (2022) Has COVID killed the medical conference? BMJ 376:o412. https://doi.org/10.1136/bmj.o412
15. Sa MJ, Ferreira CM, Serpa S (2019) Virtual and face-to-face academic conferences: comparison and potentials. J Educ Soc Res 9(2):35–47
16. Puccinelli E et al (2022) Hybrid conferences: opportunities, challenges and ways forward. bioRxiv 2022.03.18.484941; https://doi.org/10.1101/2022.03.18.484941
17. Nursing and Midwifery Council (2019) Revalidation/what you need to do. Continuing professional development. http://tinyurl.com/NMC-revalidation-cpd. Last Accessed September 2022
18. Macmillan Cancer Support Voices for the Front Line (2019). https://www.macmillan.org.uk/_images/voices-from-the-frontline-september-2019_tcm9-355168.pdf. Last Accessed September 2022
19. Dean (2020) Cancer nurses undertake compulsory training in their own time, our survey shows. Cancer Nurs Pract 19(4):8–10
20. Potter E, Taylor V (2022) Securing future cancer care. Br J Nurs 31(5):S3–S3. https://doi.org/10.12968/bjon.2022.31.5.S3
21. Gwede CK (2021) The early impact of COVID-19 on cancer education and cancer control. J Cancer Educ 36(1):1–2. https://doi.org/10.1007/s13187-020-01952-6
22. Lim KHJ, Murali K, Thorne E et al (2021) The impact of COVID-19 on oncology professionals – one year on: lessons learned from the ESMO resilience task force survey series. ESMO Open 7(1):100374

Open Access This chapter is licensed under the terms of the Creative Commons Attribution 4.0 International License (http://creativecommons.org/licenses/by/4.0/), which permits use, sharing, adaptation, distribution and reproduction in any medium or format, as long as you give appropriate credit to the original author(s) and the source, provide a link to the Creative Commons license and indicate if changes were made.

The images or other third party material in this chapter are included in the chapter's Creative Commons license, unless indicated otherwise in a credit line to the material. If material is not included in the chapter's Creative Commons license and your intended use is not permitted by statutory regulation or exceeds the permitted use, you will need to obtain permission directly from the copyright holder.

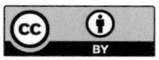

The Psychological Impact of COVID-19 on Healthcare Staff: Support Mechanisms and Leadership Approaches

9

Lucy Grant and Mark Foulkes

Check Your Experience
1. Which factors do you feel most impacted the mental health of healthcare professionals working in cancer care during the COVID-19 pandemic?
2. In your experience, which factors mitigated this impact or had the potential to do so?
3. What have we learnt from the COVID-19 pandemic in terms of supporting the mental health of healthcare professionals, which we can take forward?

Introduction

Early organisational responses to the COVID-19 pandemic were aimed at ensuring cancer services were continued for those patients with the most urgent need, whilst minimising the risk of contagion to patients, staff and society at large. It was a difficult line to tread, requiring complex planning and urgent action. In the United Kingdom, essential cancer services were protected, but there was considerable disruption to cancer care. Work practices, and the workplace itself, underwent significant change. Staff experienced redeployment, services were stepped down or suspended or delivered with reduced staffing due to sickness, some began working from home, and there was greater reliance on remote and digital technology.

Despite the amount of organisational change and the anxiety that comes from removing familiar structures and routines, this was a unique period of development, innovation and creativity. Leaders, innovators and healthcare workers came together

---

L. Grant
Berkshire Healthcare NHS Foundation Trust, Reading, Berkshire, UK
e-mail: lucy.Grant@berkshire.nhs.uk

M. Foulkes (✉)
Macmillan Lead Cancer Nurse and Nurse Consultant,
Royal Berkshire NHS Foundation Trust, Reading, UK
e-mail: mark.foulkes@royalberkshire.nhs.uk

© The Author(s) 2026
M. Foulkes et al. (eds.), *Cancer Care in the Post-COVID World*,
https://doi.org/10.1007/978-3-031-33855-7_9

to find solutions in response to the crisis. However, cancer treatment, decision-making and clinical priorities were impacted, and as a result, a backlog developed, and the impact the COVID-19 pandemic has had on patients with cancer, in the short term and long term, is considerable.

The national response to the pandemic was likened to the 'Spirit of the Blitz', and some of the rhetoric used by politicians and journalists historically evoked that used in wartime. The UK Health Secretary, Matt Hancock, called on people to emulate their grandparents' resilience during the Blitz: 'Despite the pounding every night, the rationing, the loss of life, they pulled together in a gigantic national effort. Today our generation is facing its own test, fighting a very real and new disease'. [1] Healthcare workers caring for patients with SARS-CoV-2 infection were referred to as being on the 'front line' with all staff expected to 'do one's bit'.

The wartime rhetoric was not always helpful, as Isaacs and Priesz [2] describe in their essay on the pandemic and the metaphor of war. It describes how, during the pandemic, many healthcare workers experienced a moral dilemma because 'their obligation to care for patients may conflict with their obligation to keep themselves well in order to continue caring for patients and their obligation to care for and protect their own family… healthcare workers may arguably have accepted a slightly higher risk to themselves by pursuing their vocation. While they have a duty to care for patients, they have no obligation to sacrifice themselves'. The COVID-19 pandemic highlighted a heavy moral obligation that can be placed on healthcare workers.

Delays and cancellations to treatment can greatly reduce a patient's quality of life and increase their vulnerability to stress, anxiety and depression. During the pandemic, people experienced delays to their diagnosis and restrictions to treatment, which had consequences for oncological outcomes. The impact on family members and caregivers was considerable, increasing their risk of caregiver strain and isolation [3]. How people experienced the pandemic was also influenced by their health and existing social inequalities. We have learnt from a range of studies that since the pandemic, health and social inequalities have widened [4]. SARS-CoV-2-related deaths disproportionately affected non-white ethnic groups, people with pre-existing health conditions and those dependent on care, including the elderly and people with learning disabilities living in care homes. We are still learning about the long-term and hidden consequences of the pandemic, especially on more diverse communities. 'Long COVID' is also creating many challenges in the daily activities of 1.6 million people's health, well-being and employment, which in turn further impacts the demands placed on healthcare staff [5].

The Impact of the COVID-19 Pandemic on the Mental Health of Healthcare Workers and the Psychosocial Burdens on the Cancer Workforce

The cancer workforce dealt with increasing clinical complexity and patient need at a time when they had restricted resources. Support for vulnerable and 'hard to reach' communities of patients was further limited. The impact of cancer diagnoses also increased existing vulnerability within these populations.

The cancer workforce witnessed increased mortality and morbidity, with attendant suffering and distress within the groups they were caring for. There was sustained uncertainty for people with cancer diagnoses and their families, which was further amplified by uncertainty and fragility in the health services they were relying on. These factors had a considerable impact on the mental health of the cancer workforce and posed a significant moral challenge.

This was recorded by Gilleen et al. [6] who carried out a longitudinal study surveying more than 3000 health workers in the United Kingdom during the COVID pandemic. They found that a significant proportion of health workers (28%) reported high depression, 33% reported high anxiety and 15% reported high COVID-19 pandemic-related PTSD symptoms. They also found that demographic and role-related factors were linked with clusters of symptoms. Women and frontline workers as well as those with an existing mental health disorder were more likely to report high levels of symptoms. Managers reported much higher levels of PTSD symptoms than other groups, and nurses had higher levels of symptoms than other medical staff.

Importantly, there were also found to be a number of preventable workplace factors, particularly those relating to the perception of personal risk that increased the likelihood of having high levels of PTSD symptoms. This included a pressure to reuse personal protective equipment (PPE) and a failure in workplaces to reduce risk through good preparation. Gilleen et al. concluded that the COVID-19 pandemic had a 'discernible and detrimental' effect on the mental health and well-being of health workers in the United Kingdom, but that health workers typically show low recognition of the importance of their own mental health. The study also noted that working in healthcare during a pandemic can result in long-term effects on mental health that may persist for many years.

A study by Roberts et al. [7] from Australia concentrated on the cancer workforce, with 176 healthcare workers working in oncology surveyed. They found that despite the low SARS-CoV-2 infection rates in Australia during the survey period, distress was evident in healthcare workers. The study identified the high perceived levels of responsibility that were felt for the people they cared for, the colleagues they worked with and those that lived within their families and communities.

The COVID-19 pandemic presented professional, vocational and personal challenges to healthcare workers and leaders. But it was and is remembered as a significant event and unique period in people's working lives. In the United Kingdom, in 2022, the George Cross was awarded to the four National Health Services of the United Kingdom in recognition of over 74 years of service, including the exceptional efforts of national health service (UK) (NHS) staff all across the country during the COVID-19 pandemic. The presentation was exactly one week after the NHS's birthday [8]. In the United Kingdom, the award, created in 1940 during World War II, is the highest civilian gallantry award and is equal to the military Victoria Cross: 'It is given for acts of the greatest heroism or of the most conspicuous courage in circumstances of extreme danger'.

Despite this official national honour and public recognition, the ambiguous feelings experienced and the different meanings that staff associated with the pandemic were extreme. It ranged from shock, disorientation, loss and displacement to feelings of heroism, purpose, fulfilment, engagement, determination, occupation and opportunity. We have learnt that some staff were particularly vulnerable to the adverse psychosocial consequences of the pandemic because of influences related to hierarchical position, power and social context, culture and privilege. Career stage was also a factor. For example, newly qualified staff and those approaching retirement were likely to experience more acute effects. Role longevity was another factor. For example, it was challenging if people were new to their role or had been redeployed to roles in which they had limited relevant experience. The strength of an individual's existing support structures was also relevant. It can be challenging to work with unfamiliar colleagues and to return to a team or role following a period of absence (such as a career break, maternity or sickness). It also felt challenging to be separated from loved ones and have little social and emotional support.

Staff experienced high levels of distress, emotional fatigue, exhaustion, burnout and symptoms of acute stress. Their physical, emotional and social resources were outstripped by the complex and ongoing demands of work in the face of a threatening illness and the attendant sense of uncertainty. Some staff developed the symptoms of PTSD through witnessing or experiencing traumatic and life-changing events. But we have learnt a great deal about how staff coped, the types of coping strategies they used and their individual resources. We also learnt about how that coping was influenced by their perception of risk and how they understood the level of threat. A study from Poland looked at coping strategies employed by health workers during the COVID-19 pandemic and found that the most successful strategies were those based on 'meaning-based' coping, which are strategies based on their own beliefs and values, and the existential and personal goals they use to motivate and sustain themselves. [9]

Some authors have also described 'moral injury' (MI), which is the misalignment of personal moral values and organisational approaches and structures. Moral injury occurs when an individual engages in but fails to prevent, or just witnesses, acts that conflict with their values or beliefs and when they experience betrayal by others they trust [10]. In the United Kingdom, the Welsh Government believed that MI was such a significant issue for healthcare staff during the COVID-19 pandemic that a briefing paper was published outlining strategies to address it [10]. This recognises that although MI is not a mental illness in itself, it can contribute to other mental health problems, such as PTSD. The paper gives examples where healthcare workers might experience MI, such as being present at a patient's death without loved ones present, or having to allocate limited resources to severely unwell patients, or feeling let down by others with regard to their safety. Many healthcare professionals working in oncology would have experienced the first two of these examples with increased mortality rates, the restrictions placed on visiting oncology and haematology units and the adaptations made to SACT regimens in the early days of the pandemic. In addition, the experience of limited access to PPE was catastrophically widespread in healthcare across Europe.

Healthcare systems across Europe are now addressing a vast backlog of delayed diagnoses and increasing demand from an ageing population for improved access to more effective treatments. The current exodus of staff leaving cancer services, the low levels of recruitment and increased industrial unrest linked to inadequate pay during a cost-of-living crisis can be traced, in large measure, to the frail and broken post-pandemic healthcare systems they are having to work in. A recent study by the University of Bath has shown that the most frequently reported reasons for staff leaving their jobs in the NHS are, in order of importance [11]:

1. Stress
2. Shortage of staff/resources
3. Pay

Another recent major finding is that there is strong evidence of high rates of under-reporting of important staff worries to line managers, especially with regard to the impact of mental health. There is also evidence that rates of negative impacts on well-being were greatest amongst groups who were involuntarily redeployed to SARS-CoV-2 infection care. Those groups have the highest rates of staff disposed to exit employment with the NHS, which highlights a sense of ongoing dissatisfaction and moral injury amongst them.

In the post-pandemic landscape in cancer care, it is important that the long-term psychological sequelae and key lessons of the pandemic are recognised and managed proactively. This is a key period for learning, integration and recovery. The recognition of the changes that have occurred in the workplace and working practices and the impact these have on the social and psychological elements of work are important. Monitoring for ongoing issues is priority, so interventions and support can be targeted to mitigate chronicity and the severity of psychological symptoms.

Approaches, Roles and Interventions

(a) *Compassionate Leadership and Emotional Containment*

The pandemic gave healthcare services worldwide an opportunity to consider the response to mass trauma and humanitarian crises. Narratives were essential because they weaved meaning around 'being in it together', social responsibility, cooperation and sharing experiences of pain and suffering. As we have seen, meaning-based strategies are effective in helping face adversity with compassion and determination. During the pandemic, we witnessed many social barriers breaking down and community action as our feelings of connectedness and interdependency were highlighted. The experience of those 'on the front line' and 'doing one's bit' was made visible and presented as heroes. 'Clap for heroes' was a public gesture of appreciation for health workers in the NHS, which took place every Thursday evening at 8pm between 26 March and 28 May 2020. The idea, which began in Europe, was promoted by a Dutch woman living in London, prompting politicians and celebrities to support the national campaign. But the practice of applauding was heavily criticised by many health workers as an empty gesture and political deflection amid budget cuts and PPE shortages for the NHS.

Through compassionate leadership, the collective management of meaning and communication is critical in containing the physical and psychological elements of the work. Teams that had existing and effective support and communication strategies could draw on these structures. They could stay connected to each other's experiences and be a container for the terrible suffering they were witnessing and experiencing. But for teams that were broken up, displaced or disbanded through organisational necessity, it was a far harder task. Suffering and distress were displaced and fragmented.

Local leadership and management proved crucial to managing the well-being of staff and anticipating and validating their support needs. So too was adopting a resilience framework that philosophically emphasised that emotional suffering is a natural part of living and is a normal response to loss and trauma, death and dying. The importance of compassionate leadership has been highlighted as a vital component in coping with stressful situations in healthcare. Gotsis, [12] in his study of the role of compassionate leadership in post-pandemic healthcare, points out that compassion is regarded as a cornerstone of patient-centred care in healthcare organisations and that compassionate leadership must adopt holistic and supportive strategies and shared distributive styles in order to find innovative responses to challenges. In this way, healthcare leaders and managers need to demonstrate psychological thinking to be more emotionally present to their colleagues' experiences and suffering and their role in emotional containment.

From 1959, the pioneering organisational consultant and psychoanalyst, Isabel Menzies Lyth (1917–2008), wrote her classic studies on social systems functioning as a defence against anxiety. She describes how social defences are manifest within hospital systems and healthcare settings so that staff can cope with the heightened anxiety associated with the task of caring for people that are ill and dying, including the field of cancer and palliative care nursing [13]. Her work revealed how commonplace it was for social defences to become too defensive and the culture of the hospital and its practices to lead to the disavowal of the psychological elements of caring for patients. Clinical tasks and ward routines were enforced by a rigid hierarchy and routines with strict rules that dehumanised the patient and detached nurses from the emotion of caring for patients. It stifled professional growth by preventing more mature forms of coping with anxiety from developing. Menzies Lyth explored the vital role that leadership and management have in being present to and understanding the powerful and potentially destructive organisational dynamics, so that the idea of 'defences' could be identified and then reflected upon to create systems to support staff to emotionally connect to task of caring for patients.

However, during the COVID pandemic, many senior staff, including leaders and management, were absent from the clinical environment, which greatly increased the risk that those on the front line were left alone without the support of leadership, which amplified levels of anxiety. Strauss et al. believe that the key characteristic of compassionate leadership is emotional intelligence [14]. This incorporates knowledge about emotions, using emotional skills, and an ability to apply that knowledge to emotional situations. A recent study from Finland, which took place during the COVID-19 pandemic, identified that leaders had a vital role in promoting a compassionate atmosphere [15]. Being physically present in the workplace and fostering an open dialogue amongst the working community were key to compassionate leadership. Here in the United Kingdom, the Kings Fund published a toolkit of recommendations to help nurses deliver the highest possible standard of care during the pandemic. One of its eight recommendations was to ensure that care environments had compassionate leadership and nurturing cultures that enabled both patient care and staff support to be both high quality and continually improve [16].

An important part of providing compassionate leadership is the use of effective containment and holding. As a concept, containment and holding stem from the field of psychoanalysis. This is the ability to provide a safe and supportive environment where emotions, thoughts and experiences can be expressed and then thought about and explored. In a management context, the container/containment concept refers to a leader's ability to create a safe and supportive environment where staff members can express their emotions and ideas around their work without fear of judgement or overwhelming experiences. This idea becomes particularly relevant to those working in cancer care to provide often distressed and vulnerable patients with a sense of safety by demonstrating professionalism, compassion, empathy and gentle encouragement.

Writing in 2020, Dr Catherine Sadler stated that healthcare leaders needed to take four steps to provide emotional containment for a stressed workforce [17]. These are:

1. Take prompt and visible action.
2. Engage in clear and honest communication.
3. Provide empathy and understanding.
4. Inspire through highlighting organisational strengths.

Stadler suggested that during the pandemic and continuing into the post-pandemic period, healthcare leaders would need to apply these in practice by being more transparent about what they can and cannot do, communicating more honestly, more frequently and in greater detail through various channels. They also needed to demonstrate greater empathy by acknowledging and legitimising their colleagues' experiences and providing encouragement and hope via individual success stories.

(b) *Trauma-Informed Approaches*

Supporting the workforce to meet the increasingly complex psychological needs of people with cancer and to understand the role of trauma is a strategic and operational priority. Implementation needs to be systematic and at an organisational level to ensure support is embedded within the culture of organisations. Healthcare professionals need access to up-to-date training, education, as well as clinical supervision, and reflective practice structures that include the promotion of self-care and awareness of the impact of caring on the self. This is necessary to fulfil the significant role they have in supporting patients and mitigating the psychological impact of cancer. Without adequate support mechanisms, healthcare professionals are not able to confidently and safely engage with the psychological tasks of caring for people with cancer because of risk of becoming overwhelmed.

Trauma-informed approaches aim to recognise, understand and empathise with the pervasive impact of trauma on an individual and those around them. The relevance for healthcare providers relates to the heightened risk of those with trauma having their trauma re-triggered in medical and healthcare settings. Training healthcare professionals to interact to reduce the risk of re-traumatisation helps to reduce the anxiety associated with receiving care for those with trauma [18].

In November 2022, the Health Service in the United Kingdom sought to more clearly define what trauma-informed practice entails [18]. 'Trauma-informed' approaches were being increasingly adopted as a means to reduce the impact of trauma on psychological well-being and to support mental and physical health outcomes. Trauma-informed approaches became particularly relevant during the pandemic. The Office for Health Improvement and Disparities concluded that 'trauma-informed practice is an approach to health and care interventions which is grounded in the understanding that trauma exposure can impact an individual's neurological, biological, psychological and social development'. [18]

In 2021, Fenney highlighted the importance of trauma-informed strategies in meeting the support needs of people suffering from trauma during the pandemic [19]. Her aim was to increase awareness of how trauma negatively impacts individuals and communities in their ability to feel safe. Trauma also lessens the ability to develop trusting relationships with healthcare staff and the services they provide.

Principles of trauma-informed care can equally be applied to healthcare staff working with people with cancer during the pandemic because they were exposed to vicarious trauma, secondary traumatic stress and so many experienced burnout. In 2023, Dawson-Rose et al. [20] published a plea for a trauma-informed approach to prevent burnout in nurses, which cited six principles:

1. Safety
2. Trustworthiness and transparency
3. Peer support
4. Collaboration
5. Empowerment, voice and choice
6. Moving past gender, historic and cultural issues

A trauma-informed approach that utilises all of these six principles whilst validating and promoting self-care as an essential element of how we stay healthy and effective at work is most likely to be effective. Healthcare organisations should promote proactive and routine self-care and reflective practice amongst healthcare staff working with cancer patients. People cope in different ways. Offering and signposting different types of support mechanisms is important. For example, the concept of 'psychological first aid' is helpful because it advocates that psychological safety and well-being must first prioritise primary needs such as nutrition, hygiene, personal environment and rest. Only after this has been achieved can psychological processing and restorative reflection take place.

Even though 'trauma-informed' approaches have been recommended and, in part, implemented, there may be questions raised around the extent, thoroughness and therefore quality of these approaches in a psychological sense. Embedding a thorough and effective trauma-informed system of support is highly complex and requires continuous monitoring and adjustment. Many of the systems put in place during and immediately after the COVID-19 pandemic are relatively underdeveloped and thus, as yet, unproven.

(c) *Building Resilience*

Emotional resilience is our ability to respond to stressful or unexpected situations and crises. The amount of emotional resilience we have is determined by different things, including our age, identity and what we have experienced in our lives. When individuals deal with traumatic or troubling events, emotional turbulence and higher levels of stress are normal reactions and not a sign of pathology. With proactive approaches to coping, active coping and access to timely and tailored support, these reactions can be stabilised. Even prior to the COVID-19 pandemic, there was increased focus on trying to increase the resilience of healthcare staff working in cancer care, but the pandemic has given it an urgency. In a multinational study, Cloconi et al. found that higher burnout levels were linked to lower resilience, whilst those with higher resilience had lower burnout [21]. The multinational cross-sectional study found that the most successful strategies in building resilience were adaptive coping with cognitive and behavioural efforts to manage stressful conditions; tangible instrumental support; emotional support such as encouragement, reassurance and compassion; and positive reframing of ways that a stressor may be positive or beneficial.

A Norwegian study considered the factors that drive resilience building [22]. It found that the key capacities for resilience in healthcare were leadership, structure, communication, learning, coordination, alignment, involvement, competence, effective facilitators and risk awareness. Resilience to adversity comes from how we make sense of our experiences and who helps to do so. One of the most important factors is to have clear and accessible lines of communication with colleagues. Ideally, there should be a facilitated structure that encourages the sharing of tolerant, enriching and inclusive narratives about overcoming adversity, which supports and respects people's feelings and different coping mechanisms and within which they feel safe enough to show their distress and vulnerability.

Implications

The long-term implications of the psychological impact of the pandemic on the cancer care workforce across Europe have yet to be fully understood. The workplace and working practices have changed significantly and continue to do so. The direct psychological trauma, moral challenges and ongoing uncertainty have all had an impact on healthcare workers, individually and collectively. Multiple studies from across Europe and elsewhere have reported increased rates of depression, anxiety, stress and post-traumatic stress disorder (PTSD) compared to pre-pandemic levels. 'Compassion fatigue', 'burnout' and 'moral injury' are frequently reported by healthcare staff, and the evidence suggests that this has led to more staff choosing to leave health services or considering doing so [11]. In addition to the purely psychological impacts of exposure to harm during the COVID-19 pandemic, we do not yet fully understand the impact on overall health of 'Long-COVID', and this may combine with mental health issues to further disrupt and deplete the cancer-care workforce [23].

As Europe continues to adapt to the post-pandemic landscape, healthcare systems have learnt that there needs to be closer attention to the mental well-being of their staff. Considering the social and psychological experience of staff becomes more important with the use of digital technology and the increase in remote working practices. There is little doubt that as time goes on, strategies in cancer care and other specialities will need to adapt and develop support mechanisms and leadership approaches to promote staff well-being to avoid healthcare staff shortages with resultant poor outcomes for patients.

COVID-19 has encouraged us to rethink what we already knew about the role of leadership and acknowledge the psychological elements of healthcare. Healthcare organisations where leaders promote inclusiveness, collaboration and diversity, prioritise staff well-being and embed an array of supportive structures and mechanisms will be more resilient.

References

1. Bagehot (2020) Spirit of the blitz: history is a valuable resource in dark times, March 21st 2020, The Economist
2. Isaacs D, Priesz A (2021) COVID-19 and the metaphor of war. J Paediatr Child Health 57(1):6–8
3. Macmillan Cancer Support (2020) The forgotten C: the impact of Covid-19 on cancer care. Macmillan Cancer Support. https://www.macmillan.org.uk/dfsmedia/1a6f23537f7f4519bb0cf14c45b2a629/9601-10061/the-forgotten-c-the-impact-of-covid-on-cancer-care. Last accessed June 2023
4. Eurofound (2023) Economic and social inequalities in Europe in the aftermath of the COVID-19 pandemic. Publications Office of the European Union, Luxembourg. https://www.eurofound.europa.eu/sites/default/files/ef_publication/field_ef_document/ef22002en.pdf. Last accessed June 2023
5. Waitzman E (2022) Long COVID: what are the short- and long-term challenges? UK Parliament, House of Lords Library. https://lordslibrary.parliament.uk/long-covid-what-are-the-short-and-long-term-challenges/#heading-2. Last accessed July 2023
6. Gilleen J et al (2021) Impact of the COVID-19 pandemic on the mental health and well-being of UK healthcare workers. BJPsych (Open) 7(e88):1–12
7. Roberts NA et al (2022) From doctors to ancillary staff: regional and metropolitan cancer workforce perceptions and distress resulting from COVID-19 pandemic adaptations. Semin Oncol 49(6):490–496

8. NHS England (2022) NHS staff honoured with George Cross presentation. https://www.england.nhs.uk/2022/07/nhs-staff-honoured-with-george-cross-presentation/. Last accessed June 2023
9. Krok D, Zarzycka B (2020) Risk perception of COVID-19, meaning-based resources and psychological well-being amongst healthcare personnel: the mediating role of coping. J Clin Med 9(10):3225
10. Communication and Behavioural Insights Sub-group (2021) Technical Advisory Group: moral injury in healthcare workers during the COVID-19 pandemic. Lyywodreath Cymru (Welsh Government). https://www.gov.wales/technical-advisory-group-moral-injury-health-care-workers-during-covid-19-pandemic-html. Last accessed May 2023
11. Weyman A et al (2023) Should I stay or should I go? NHS staff retention in the post COVID-19 world: challenges and prospects. IPR report. University of Bath, UK. https://www.bath.ac.uk/publications/should-i-stay-or-should-i-go-nhs-staff-retention-in-the-post-covid-19-world/attachments/NHS-staff-retention-IPR-report.pdf. Last accessed May 2023.
12. Gotsis G (2022) Leading with compassion: how compassion can enrich healthcare leadership in a post-COVID-19 world. In: Virtues and leadership: understanding and practicing good leadership. Taylor and Francis, London
13. Menzies IEP (1959) The functioning of social systems as a defence against anxiety. Hum Relat 13:95–121; Menzies IEP (1960) A case-study in the functioning of social systems as a defence against anxiety: a report on a study of the nursing service of a general hospital. Hum Relat 13(2):95–121. See also: Lyth (1988) Isabel containing anxiety in institutions: selected essays. Free Association Books, London
14. Strauss C, Lever Taylor B, Gu J, Kuyken W, Baer R, Jones et al (2016) What is compassion and how can we measure it? A review of definitions and measures. Clin Psychol Rev 47:15–27
15. Salminen-Tuomaala MH, Seppala S (2021) 'Nurses' experiences and expectations for compassionate leadership and compassion in the working community – a qualitative study. Research Square. https://doi.org/10.21203/rs.3.rs-686353/v1. Last accessed June 2023.
16. West M, Bailey S, Williams E (2020) The courage of compassion: supporting nurses and midwives to deliver high-quality care. The Kings Fund UK. www.kingsfund.org.uk/compassion. Last accessed June 2023
17. Sadler C (2020) Can healthcare leaders provide emotional containment for their staff as COVID-19 levels fall? BMJ Leader Blog, June 3. https://blogs.bmj.com/bmjleader/2020/06/03/can-healthcare-leaders-provide-emotional-containment-for-their-staff-as-covid-19-levels-fall-by-catherine-sandler/. Last accessed June 2023
18. Office for Health Improvement and Disparities (2022) Working definition of trauma-informed practice. UK Government. https://www.gov.uk/government/publications/working-definition-of-trauma-informed-practice/working-definition-of-trauma-informed-practice. Last accessed June 2023
19. Fenney D (2021) The role of trauma-informed care during the Covid-19 pandemic. The Kings Fund UK. https://www.kingsfund.org.uk/blog/2021/04/role-trauma-informed-care-covid-19. Last accessed June 2023
20. Dawson-Rose C, Cuca Y, Kumar S, Collins A (2023) Using a trauma-informed approach to address burnout in nursing: what an organization can accomplish. OJIN 28(1):1
21. Cloconi C, Economou M, Charalambous A (2023) Burnout, coping and resilience of the cancer care workforce during the SARS-CoV-2: a multinational cross-sectional study. Eur J Oncol Nurs 63:102204
22. Lyng HB, Macrae C, Guise V et al (2021) Capacities for resilience in healthcare; a qualitative study across different healthcare contexts. BMC Health Serv Res 22:474
23. Kluge, Hans Henri P (2023) Statement – 36 million people across the European Region may have developed long COVID over the first 3 years of the pandemic. https://www.who.int/europe/news/item/27-06-2023-statement%2D%2D-36-million-people-across-the-european-region-may-have-developed-long-covid-over-the-first-3-years-of-the-pandemic. Last accessed 27 June 2023

Open Access This chapter is licensed under the terms of the Creative Commons Attribution 4.0 International License (http://creativecommons.org/licenses/by/4.0/), which permits use, sharing, adaptation, distribution and reproduction in any medium or format, as long as you give appropriate credit to the original author(s) and the source, provide a link to the Creative Commons license and indicate if changes were made.

The images or other third party material in this chapter are included in the chapter's Creative Commons license, unless indicated otherwise in a credit line to the material. If material is not included in the chapter's Creative Commons license and your intended use is not permitted by statutory regulation or exceeds the permitted use, you will need to obtain permission directly from the copyright holder.

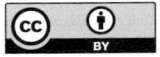

Guilt and Miracles: A Personal History of the Nightingale Hospital

10

Eamonn Sullivan

Test Your Experience
1. Leadership: From this chapter—what are the leadership lessons you have observed and could apply in your own practice?
2. Oncology contribution: What unique skills did oncology professionals bring to this endeavour?
3. Personal reflection: What would you have done differently if you were faced with such a professional and leadership challenge?

Introduction… and a Legacy

'You should be ashamed; you were the reason we had no PPE and no drugs at my hospital'!

This was VE day, May 2020, and the first time I'd felt normal in nearly three months. I'd just returned from a socially distanced street party with good friends, and as my wife and two young children walked past a group enjoying their own street party, a woman whom I'd never met came up to me saying, 'I recognise you—are you the Chief Nurse of the Nightingale?' I said yes, and the tirade began; her anger was palpable and I was stunned.

Two years later, November 2022, I was attending an 'equality in the National Health Service (NHS)' lecture with a national leader in this field—'the Nightingale Hospital is a great example of a lack of diversity and equality', the presenter stated. This was, and still is, a fraction *of* the emotion attached to 'the Nightingales', and there is no doubt that the hospitals will continue to provoke emotion, controversy and comment for some time to come. For some in the media and elsewhere, they remain highly political, 'a waste of money, a distraction or a political show', but for

E. Sullivan (✉)
New Hospital Programme, NHS England, London, UK
e-mail: eamonn.sullivan1@nhs.net

© The Author(s) 2026
M. Foulkes et al. (eds.), *Cancer Care in the Post-COVID World*,
https://doi.org/10.1007/978-3-031-33855-7_10

those of us thrown together at the start, mostly strangers, we had a simple mission on a massive scale—to save as many Londoners' lives as we could.

This chapter will tell the story of Nightingale London and the impact of cancer clinicians and cancer leaders on that endeavour.

Beginnings

I was the chief nurse at the Royal Marsden, a specialist cancer hospital in Central London, UK. This was my first chief nurse post, and I was 3 years in. I loved my job. I felt the luckiest person in the world when I was appointed. Cancer nursing fascinates and inspires me—in my opinion it is the fastest-moving area of healthcare and probably the only speciality whereby the majority of treatment modalities could completely change within the next 10 years. My clinical career had been in adult critical care, NHS and military. I am an army medical services reservist and have led Military Critical Care Teams in Iraq and Afghanistan. I had the unusual privilege of designing and opening the intensive care unit (ICU) at Camp Bastion in Helmand Province, the busiest trauma hospital in the world. It had five ICU beds.

With the Nightingale Hospital London, the mission we were given was to build the largest ICU in the world and the largest ever built, with 4000 ICU beds.

I didn't really know this at the time, but it transpired I had an unusual skill set being an NHS executive director, a board member in an Outstanding Trust, 18 years as an ICU nurse, and an army reserve officer with operational experience in austere environments.

In March 2020, we could read the signals, the first pandemic in 100 years was coming, and it was deadly. This point was clearly made when the ICU clinical director and matron emailed me a letter from the Italian Intensive Care Society. This was an open letter to ICU clinicians in Europe, and it told us to get ready as we had just weeks. It was catastrophic and I felt numb and scared. I knocked on our chief medical officer's, our chief operating officer's and chief executive's doors as we needed to dial up our plans quickly. This could potentially wipe out many of our patients, and we doubled our planning and effort to prepare. I contacted the commanding officer of my Army Reserve Unit. The colonel was a regular army officer and probably the most experienced medical logistic officer in the British Army; I had served under him in Iraq, during a particularly violent period of that war; and I had enormous respect for the man. I asked if he would provide a closed and private session for the senior leadership at the Marsden. I asked him talk about distributed leadership, a command and communication structure and supporting our staff. He attended the Marsden the next day. His session was powerful and immensely useful. Halfway through he took a call, at the end of the session—he took me aside and said, 'something huge is about to happen in London', and I said, 'Give me a call if you need anything'.

The next day I received a call from the chief nursing officer for London, asking if I would attend an urgent meeting the following day.

I was quite nervous as I entered the boardroom at Great Ormond Street Hospital in Central London. I immediately recognised my commanding officer and a colleague that I worked with in intensive care who was now the chief executive of a major London trust. There were other NHS leaders in the room, mixed with uniformed members of the military, engineers and others. The NHS chief executive for London entered and told us that London was 4000 ventilated ICU beds short, and we needed to build the world's biggest intensive care unit. He looked around the room and said we were the team that was going to do it.

We got to work immediately, and I found myself in a room with a management consultant and two medical directors, both of whom were anaesthetists. The management consultant asked, 'What is an intensive care bed? What equipment is there by each bed?' I drew a stick man and all the equipment needed around one bed. He took this, and half an hour later, he returned with a spreadsheet scaled up to 4000 ICU beds, we validated this, and he left to procure the items.

The rest of the day continued at this pace with people looking at the clinical model and considering what this would look like in terms of environment. I stressed that we needed wherever possible to reduce the physical and cognitive load on the ICU nurses and doctors, as these would be the limiting factors.

Essentially, the design was a scaled-up British Army Field hospital, a Nightingale-type environment built for reducing cognitive load and maximising visibility by one or two clinicians on the highest number of patients. This was done in a considered manner, but at a massive pace.

At the end of our meeting, one of the anaesthetists said to me, 'Eamonn, I've just been told I'm the medical director of this hospital & they have asked if you will be the chief nurse?' I responded that I would be, but I needed to check with my chief executive first. She said, 'Absolutely. Do what you need to do'.

That is the way it was with no time for niceties. We had a critical mission, and we understood the significance of what we were about to do. We did what we could.

We regrouped in the afternoon and presented our plans on the clinical model, workforce, procurement and physical environment. There was a discussion about what we should call this hospital. Would it be 'Pandemic Hospital Number One?' or 'The NHS Excel'? One of my colleagues, the new designated chief operating officer for our endeavour, suggested that, as 2020 was the year of the nurse, we should call this the 'Nightingale Hospital London'. She went on to say that Nightingale gave hope to the British public during the Crimean War and that we had that same responsibility now—to give hope to the people of London. There was total silence. Everybody agreed, and so the first of the Nightingale hospitals began.

For a group who had never met, we achieved a huge amount in one day. We finished about 10pm, and I was high on adrenaline. I went back to my hotel room, feeling emotionally and physically exhausted. It had felt like a mock tabletop exercise, but the enormity of what we were doing hit me like a steam train, and I felt quite emotional. That evening I had my first Zoom call of the pandemic with friends, everyone was in good spirits, but my mind was on the next day.

The next day we presented to the offices of a management consultancy in Canary Wharf. There we now have maybe 30 or 40 military, civilian, NHS managers, consultants, architects and other experts. I was now in my military uniform. The atmosphere felt quite different. There was certainly fear in the room. I had only seen and felt this level of fear previously when I'd served in Iraq. Fear is a unique emotion, which needs respect. You must call out, manage it, or it becomes highly destructive.

The chief operating officer, the medical director, military commander and I were asked to go into the centre of the room to 'calm the nerves'. People were pacing, anxious and scared, and the fear was palpable. Our brilliant chief operating officer (only appointed the previous evening) walked straight into the centre of the room and 'called out' the fear in one of the best leadership moments I have ever seen in my career. She read the room perfectly, turned and looked at everybody and said, 'It's okay to be frightened'. Complete silence. 'We are all scared but we are the team that is going to deliver this hospital for Londoners, and we will support each other through this'. The medical director and military commander said equally inspiring words whilst I looked at people in the room and said, 'Some of us are going to get sick and that is okay. If you are feeling unwell, please tell us. We will take you off the pitch, we will look after you and get you back in the fight again if you want to'. The tension was eased, people were focused, and we got to work continuing the work that we had started the previous day but at an increased pace.

We were told that the Nightingale Hospital was confirmed to be in London's Excel Exhibition Centre and that we would start work on site the next day.

The Vision

That second afternoon, a small group of us, key management consultants, our chief operating officer, medical director, clinical leads, military commander and myself, sat in a room.

- We knew that this would be the most challenging piece of work that our people would ever do in their lives; we also knew that the stress on the caregivers would be overwhelming and unprecedented. We were looking at potentially a six-to-ten nurse-patient ratio which carried a high risk. People would die, but our job was to ensure that most people lived. We knew we would be doing things never done in the history of the NHS or indeed in the history of healthcare. We needed a vision and some simple messaging for all staff. We came up with some principles.
- Our first principle was simple: *to save Londoners' lives*.
- Secondly, we pledged that *nobody would die alone*, and that we would do everything humanly possible to ensure that the dying would have their family beside them on the intensive care unit, regardless of the PPE and staffing challenges.
- This was an extremely high-risk project—so critical would be to build an innovative 'learning system' to '*make each day better than yesterday*'. We had to learn very quickly to keep patients and staff safe.

- Most importantly I believed we needed to *'treat our people like rock stars'* for example, if a staff nurse's grandmother needed a pint of milk, we would get them a pint of milk to her doorstep that same day. We would wrap around the most advanced welfare system in the NHS around our staff. We changed the paradigm from the patient being in the centre to the patient and the caregiver in the centre, with services rotating around them ensuring the best possible outcome for both.

Operations

The Excel Conference Centre in East London would deliver healthcare on a scale never seen. It had a corridor (or 'spine'), the width of a motorway down the centre, a kilometre long. Straddling this spine were two massive halls—the South and North Hall. Each hall was the size and length of six full football pitches back to back, and our plan was to put 2000 ICU beds in each of these halls.

On the third planning day, we again split into a group: workforce, procurement, clinical model, management, model and environment build. It was beginning to take shape. Healthcare architects began doing the drawings there and then.

What I now needed most was a clinical leadership team, clinical experts in critical care nursing and therapies, but these staff were in very high demand. I made contact with the brilliant chief nurse for London, and everyone else in my phone book. I even phoned the chief therapist for England directly one Sunday morning asking for help; I appreciated that critical care therapists would be crucial to the success of the endeavour. I had a mixed response, hospitals were under massive pressure, and many had opened 'augmented care areas' and had scores of ventilated patients well above their 'pre-Covid' numbers. One chief nurse asked, 'What are you doing, Eamonn? We can't help'. That response particularly deflated me as I was really relying on that particular team, and she had said categorically 'no'. The next morning in walked a team from this particular teaching hospital, an elite team of the best critical care, nurses and therapists from that hospital and I felt elated.

We had just days to open the unit, and 48 h later, the Excel looked completely different. There were hundreds of staff building the ICU; these were a mixture of 'events' experts who would normally be building exhibitions in the Excel, combined with hundreds of soldiers, working under their supervision. The change was remarkable as they worked around the clock.

I called upon colleagues in the Royal Marsden Hospital. Within a week two oncology ICU matrons, the leading acute physician and the hospital's chief pharmacist, arrived at the Excel to be part of the leadership team. In terms of the size of the Marsden, this was a disproportionately high number of key clinical leaders, and the flexibility and adaptability of cancer clinicians would soon become apparent.

As a senior leadership team, we were becoming anxious. The Grenfell Tower public inquiry was deliberating, and many of the public service leaders involved in that tragedy were under scrutiny, and it was difficult to watch; careers and livelihoods were being destroyed. A small group of us were taking on this massive responsibility which we did so readily—but we also were cognisant of the risks in which if this were to go wrong, it might be on a scale never seen before in the United Kingdom or the world. We needed advice and air cover to be able to perform, or we would collapse under the stress and be unable to make the decisions that were required. For example, we were acutely aware that even with contingency planning, a fire, oxygen or electrical failure in a facility would be catastrophic and was a terrifying prospect. The NHS leaders organised for a QC judge, an expert in public enquiries, to come and speak to us in a closed session about what the aftermath could look like—even in the worst case, and including the inevitable public enquiry, this gave us a lot of strength, put what we were doing in context and was a useful caveat to building our own personal resilience to be able to carry on and take the very high-risk decisions that we had to take. There could be no hesitation.

We had many VIP visits in the first nine days leading up to us opening. One in particular left a lasting impact on me, and that was one of the national professional leads stepping into the cavernous empty hall with me. She knew what we were about to do and facing into. We both welled up. This national lead was one of a small number who worked with us throughout, on a weekly basis, alongside us and in other ICUs. She said that she could not advocate for us on a national level if she did not understand what it was really like at the bedside in an ICU or ward in a pandemic.

Work intensified as we neared the day nine opening, and there was much media interest. We engaged with local intensive care units and health leaders to get staff released from various units in London—which themselves were under massive pressure.

We also worked with small teams of empowered staff or 'fixers'. These were capable clinical and non-clinical people, mostly not from an ICU background, whom we would give 'problems to solve'. These roles were invaluable, allowing us to move at pace and not be slowed or distracted by knotty problems that needed solutions before the unit opened. For example, wayfinding within such a huge environment was difficult. One team produced the entire wayfinding and naming strategy within one day. This was agreed and implemented the following day. Other innovations included pre-made medications to support bedside staff, methods of identifying staff roles when everyone was in blue, calling for emergency assistance, managing security, checking in and handover, safety messaging, admitting, tracking patients, communicating with family members and many other small but essential 'problems' solved by our 'fixer' teams.

We paid significant attention to our communication structures from the outset. In such a large and new organisation, effective communication is absolutely critical. Our objective was to ensure staff felt safe to speak out and speak up but especially to feel part of what we were doing. They needed to feel that they could influence our direction and not just be passive caregivers or managers, but respected partners in this high-risk endeavour. We wanted our staff to tell their story and to look back on this as one of the most prominent and positive experiences of their careers, despite the stress and risk.

To do so, as a leadership team, we needed to keep very close to our people and to be highly visible at all times. We analysed the cadence of the 24-h cycle of the unit and put in touch points with staff throughout that period. Some were planned, and some organic, according to the needs at that time. We knew that we would be in the media spotlight externally, but we were also aware that it would be impossible to completely control the social media narrative with such a large number of staff who were highly digital and social media savvy. From the outside, we did not put restrictions on social media use other than well-established protocols that clinical staff were familiar with. As a leadership team, we observed and interacted with staff's personal social media feeds, looking on the medium as an important form of staff feedback. We also tested and deployed innovative apps such as the brilliant 'Improvewell' which is a clever app combining health and well-being with feedback—so staff could access help on their terms and feel more part of the mission.

This blending of traditional communication methods with the staff's organic use of social media, both as a platform to tell their story and also relieve stress, meant that, with some exceptions, the narrative was appropriate, giving the public confidence and our staff freedom to express their lived experience in such unprecedented times.

We opened on time and the first desperately Ill patients arrived. Within a short period, 35 ventilated Londoners were being cared for in a conference hall in East London to the same standard as local intensive care units. This was, we believe, the largest temporary ICU in Europe.

At the height of the endeavour, over 600 staff lived in hotels around the Excel facility. Some lived there for weeks or months on end, away from their families and loved ones. As part of our staff well-being and welfare offer, we used established protocols from our military colleagues, that is, the same principles the Armed Forces use to support their staff when they are overseas on operations. The goal here was for staff to be freed up from the 'distractions and stresses' of everyday life so they could focus on being an ICU nurse, an ICU physiotherapist, cleaning manager or other role. What this practically meant was that we provided free accommodation on site, laundry, Internet, hot food around the clock, access to quiet areas, access to healthcare, barbers, a small grocery shop, travel and all the 'physical' things that we could do to relieve staff from those daily tasks—so they could focus on providing care to Londoners or having proper downtime with their new colleagues or on their own. Like many NHS hospitals at that time, we were overwhelmed by the kindness of members of the public and the local community, who were very generous and went above and beyond to look after our staff and their local community.

As well as physical well-being, we paid as much attention to psychological well-being. Using a blended military and civilian approach, staff had access to around-the clock support. This started with self-help, buddy-buddy support and access to trained volunteers, right the way through to the best military psychiatrists and military mental health nurses on site.

Team composition was crucially important. We had staff from over 30 hospitals who came together at no notice to provide high-risk critical care in a conference centre in East London. How teams were composed, how they were led, the shift patterns that they worked were all carefully considered. For example, if 12 clinical staff came from one hospital, we would work closely with them to ensure that shift patterns aligned and that they weren't all split up, plus any additions to that team were thoughtfully integrated and supported. This work happened at a rapid pace and was under constant evaluation.

Staff were highly motivated; we attempted to empower and involve them as key partners in this mission, as opposed to 'temporary' clinicians working shift by shift. Being involved and respected was crucial to their overall well-being and long-term recovery from this experience. We actively sought staff views, and often teams could see their recommendations rapidly deployed in practice the very next day or have it fed back in near real time or why the suggestion wasn't used at this particular time. This high level of staff engagement and involvement throughout was a key element in our overall aim to create a genuine culture of safety for both patients and staff.

Upon reflection, we paid as much attention to staff experience as we did to patient safety. For example, if staff members' pay was delayed or incorrect, then that would provoke the same reaction from our senior HR and management teams as a patient safety incident would for our clinical and governance teams. This attention to detail for staff experience was an enormous commitment from HR and finance teams who were dealing with multiple trusts and different systems on an unprecedented scale.

At any one time, more than one hundred of these staff from cleaning or catering staff to doctors, nurses and therapists would present each shift. The logistics of coordinating such a roster was immense. Staffing was a constant pinch point, and a large, dedicated team were tasked with recruiting, training, allocating and supporting these staff. We had multiple daily meetings with the health system in London looking at capacity and demand, transferring patients in and out to support the needs of London. Our major limiting factor was staff, as was the case in most ICUs at that time.

We had an expert multi-professional education training and orientation team. They were based at 'The O2', the massive music concert arena in South London. They mocked up an exact replica of the intensive care unit and trained thousands of staff from all disciplines in ICU clinical care logistics management. The Nightingale was, and still is, the longest-standing event at The O2. For just over 44 days, the education and onboarding team prepared staff to work, not just in the Nightingale, but in hospitals across London.

We developed new staffing models to affirm our ethos of reducing the physical and psychological cognitive load from the bedside staff and support our clinicians to do what only they could to work only at the top of their licence. To achieve this, we developed new models of care focusing on what tasks needed to be done per patient, per cohort of patients or per unit of patients. We looked at the skills of different clinicians, as we had many anaesthetists, but few intensivists; we maximised the use of the intensivists by freeing them up from certain tasks that anaesthetists were very comfortable with, such as the insertion of central venous and arterial lines. We developed 'line teams' whose task was to insert lines each shift. We also developed physiotherapy led 'proning teams', mixtures of clinical and non-clinical staff, to prone and un-prone patients safely.

We knew that ICU nurses would be the scarcest resource, so we developed personal hygiene teams, IV medicine teams and others to free up the ICU nurses from certain physical tasks. This type of innovation was happening all over the NHS at rapid speed. We developed many of the protocols and shared these across the NHS.

We started with a nurse-to-patient ratio of 1 to 6 ventilated patients, which was the ratio used in many of the hospitals in London in the first few weeks of the pandemic; this quickly fell to 1 to 4 and then 1 to 2. We used others, community nurses, therapists, volunteer ambulance staff and medics to work with the ICU nurses to ensure that every patient had a member of staff attending to them.

These new ways of working required new ways of training and educating our staff. For example, the ICU nurse pre-pandemic was used to caring for just one or two ventilated patients. We were asking them to be a conductor and positioned them in the centre of four or six patients—and coordinating the care by working through others at the bedside. This was a new way of working for many of these young ICU nurses, so we had to train them in how to conduct and coordinate care at a different level. This was done through our education 'onboarding' team who developed new protocols. We had many oncology nurses, and in my experience, they proved highly adaptable and agile despite working in such an uncertain and different environment; the cancer nurses' confidence with complex medicines was a huge asset. Their expertise in communicating with family members was invaluable. Their expertise in end-of-life care was called upon to train and support other team members.

With such pressures working in the facility was an intense experience for the staff. The central spine of the Excel was a preserved clean area. The main life support for the hospital was housed here such as the hospital management cell, stores, pharmacy, health and well-being, handover and other critical infrastructure in this kilometre-long spine. Entering the actual intensive care unit was an austere experience, made easier by the kindness and compassion of the Virgin cabin crew and St John Ambulance volunteers who supported staff donning their PPE and preparing to enter the dirty area, the actual intensive care unit. Walking onto the unit was surreal, vision was obstructed, breathing was difficult, everybody was in blue. To the non-critical care eye, it was a chaotic scene, but it was actually highly organised and coordinated in every detail. Thinking about that sight, even now, literally takes my breath away. More than 30 patients, nearly all people of colour, were proned, ventilated, unconscious and desperately unwell. London's finest security guards, bus drivers, nurses and building workers all were critically ill and totally dependent on the expertise and care of strangers to survive.

Bedside staff cared for patients up to 4 h at a time. They were then rotated out to the well-being area for a rest. Here the volunteers ensured that the staff had what they needed to take some time out before re-entering the unit and continuing with their shift. Of course, such scenes were playing out in intensive care unit across the whole of England and indeed the world. What made it very different for us was that we were in a conference centre in East London miles from any actual hard-standing hospital.

We kept true to our pledge to ensure that the dying always had a member of their family with them; this was a challenge as like many units, we often had severe shortages of PPE. The chaplains from all faiths were amazing. They coordinated this effort to support the dying 24 h a day, 7 days a week. Cancer nurses and doctors remained instrumental in the care of the dying and delivering advanced communication with family members, supporting the strategic effort across London, as well as the operational and tactical bedside response in many units.

As the director of nursing, I had a number of different commitments; I was a member of the executive board of the Nightingale, working closely with the team from St Bartholomew's Hospital (Barts') whom we were under the professional and leadership umbrella of. This relationship was really important; it allowed us to have full access to the resources of the Barts' campuses including clinical governance, information and computing, facilities and workforce. We could also 'be in step' with Barts' in terms of escalation and de-escalation of staffing ratios and other clinical ICU protocols and standard operating procedures. This was, in my opinion, crucial for the safe running of the Nightingale and integration into the wider London health system.

As the weeks went on, we found that we had become, by default, the Nightingale 'experts'—and our skills were called upon to support other organisations establish Nightingale Hospitals in England, Scotland and Wales. We were the only Nightingale to be fully operational and care for ICU patients.

In terms of my own team of senior nurses, therapists and pharmacists, we soon got into a 'daily battle rhythm', whereby we would meet several times a day. I set out from the beginning to put trust at the centre of my own personal leadership style. My expectation was that this trust would be two-way and honoured, and in doing so, I shared all the inner workings of the Nightingale with my direct line reports, the coming and goings and the tactical, strategic and political elements of the endeavour. Nothing was off the table. This sense of trust and openness strengthened our bond together and the feeling that we were all in this as one and that everyone had a voice and would be heard. There were no games, no egos, we had to be open and supportive with each other. I also invested time at the beginning to get to know each of them. We were thrown together, and I needed to know what each of their professional and personal worries and fears were, so I could support them in the extremely high stress and responsibility that they were carrying on a daily basis. Theirs was a physically and psychologically demanding job—working day and night shifts as the senior clinical leaders on the floor. I had and still have enormous respect for them all.

Patient safety was our number one priority, and we sought always 'to do no harm'. The patient safety and governance model were the centrepiece of the operational phase of the Nightingale Hospital. Our improvement and learning model aimed to really *'make tomorrow better than today,'* and we were fortunate to have some of the brightest improvement and patient safety minds in our leadership teams. At the core of patient safety was a staff culture of openness and transparency. Like all ICUs, things will and did go wrong, and we were committed to taking swift action to minimise harm to patients. At the core of the safety and learning system was a 4 pm huddle each day in which 60–80 people would participate—the brief would observe what worked well, what the external evidence was telling about the disease, what near misses or incidents had occurred and what actions we needed to take.

We found that by having the right people in the room to inform decisions, collocated beside the actual decision makers, we dramatically cut down decision, action and feedback cycles. Work was split into 'fix now', 'delegate' or 'escalate'—with most patient safety and experience actions falling into the 'fix now' box. This added to the staff involvement and empowerment elements described above. There was a team of 'bedside learning coordinators' who swept the intensive care unit, looking for near misses, actual harm and immediate feedback from bedside staff. We fed these into the 4 o'clock all-hands huddle striving always to make tomorrow better than today.

As days turned into weeks, what became apparent was that SARS-CoV-2 infection was not a single organ disease. The virus was inflicting terrible damage across multiple organs, and patients were desperately sick. Cardiac arrhythmias, strokes, kidney failure and many other conditions came to the fore. Our brilliant academics worked with local, national and international leaders to ensure that we were providing the latest evidence-based care; sometimes this was changing daily.

A key facet of our original clinical model was to decompress London intensive care units that may become saturated with Covid-positive ICU patients. Toward the end of April, London was coping with the Covid pandemic and coping very well. The need for ventilating large numbers of patients in a conference *centre* thankfully appeared to be waning. This was hugely positive news for our entire team and led to discussions within the senior health leaders regarding suspending the Nightingale Hospital London. Through the use of data and discussion, the appropriate decision was taken to hibernate Nightingale London with immediate effect. The final ventilated patients were transferred out of the facility, and intense work began to 'put Nightingale to sleep'.

Hibernating the Nightingale took several weeks and was surprisingly as intensive as setting her up. Once again, the military minds were essential in this element of the endeavour. The military is used to setting up and carefully putting away temporary field hospitals. We had to very carefully reverse engineer the set-up process—archive all of the learning, the environment and workforce models and all protocols and operating processes, so any team could come back in and set up the Nightingale once again and do so in a matter of hours or days. The NHS wanted us to retain some ventilated and ward capacity for London for the inevitable wave 2. This process took us well into May 2020.

Ending Well

There remained a high level of anxiety and activity right up until the very last patient was transferred out to a major London teaching hospital. This patient was desperately unwell, and the transfer was high risk; however, they were successfully transferred by our senior team, including one of our Nightingale medical directors who was an ICU professor.

Concurrent to the hibernation efforts, our chief operating officer was determined that the project should 'end well' for the hundreds of staff who invested so much over the previous three months, indeed, some living on site for weeks or months on end.

A late-night meeting with our most experienced 'fixer team' solidified the action. We were to organise a physical debriefing for 700 staff, face to face in one day whilst adhering to the strict lockdown and infection prevention laws of the day. This was typical 'Nightingale' scale of ambition, drive and delivery. We also deployed an amazing human asset pool that had recently come on board, a group of NHS graduate trainees from a wide range of NHS disciplines such as human resources, finance, operations and education. These 'fresh-legs' young people were a huge 'force multiplier'—an accelerant for our 'fixer team' who had worked non-stop for nearly 8 weeks.

We still 'had the keys' to the O2, which was entering its sixth week as education and simulation centre for our and London's NHS staff; at that stage, nearly 3000 staff had been through its processes and been trained. The venue was big enough to house two sittings to support 700 staff, morning and afternoon with 350 people in each cohort, socially distanced and being split up and led through four stations, each housing nearly 100 persons in huge auditoriums deep in the O2. The stations incorporated a debriefing station, a 'capturing the learning' station, a 'memorial station' and 'a thank you and next steps' station led by London and national leaders. This day was a 'closed' event and the only time in the entire endeavour that we stated to staff that there should be strictly no social media or mainstream media. This was 'private time' for staff to debrief and say goodbye to each other in a safe and spectacular environment. Despite the scale, the day felt strangely intimate and was highly emotional for many.

The O2 day was an important closure and was well evaluated. It was also a time to complete essential administration, as many of these staff remained 'on notice' to be mobilised should the need arise with the expected wave 2 of the pandemic.

Top three learning points from this chapter:

1. *A new model of care: placing care staff at the centre with the patient on an equal footing*

    I believe that the work done at the Nightingale represented an innovative shift in the model of care, rapidly pivoting away from just placing the patient at the centre of the model of care to placing the patient and the caregiver (from nurse to cleaner) at the centre together, with all support and leadership services rotating around the patient and care staff equally. As an example, in practice, as well as prioritising the holistic needs of the patient, staff needs were prioritised—whether this meant food around the clock, access to accommodation, prompt payment or ensuring that rosters were equitable with adequate rest periods between shifts. This model has particular relevance to oncology nursing, as the need to attract and retain staff by focusing on their health, well-being and work-life balance takes a more central stage.

2. *Failing fast and learning fast: embracing an improvement and staff involvement culture*

   Endeavours like the Nightingale are incredibly high risk. Failures will occur—from both a clinical and a staff welfare point of view. 'Failing fast and learning fast' was a key strategy for our leadership and clinical teams. Truly focusing 'on making tomorrow better than today' by:
   (a) Shortening communication lines
   (b) Flattening the hierarchy so all staff had a voice directly to the leadership team
   (c) Creating a culture whereby staff feel safe to report near misses, incidents and good news stories—where they feel empowered and listened to and, as a consequence, directly involved in the overall mission progression and objectives. Oncology care can particularly benefit from this approach—the care given is often not without risk in an increasingly frail and elderly population—learning quickly and applying improvement techniques to improve each day are highly relevant in cancer care.

3. *Being courageous: knowing when and how to escalate*

   As the weeks drew on, it became apparent to the Nightingale Leadership Team that London was adequately coping with the influx of wave 1 Covid patients; this coincided with the gradual fall in the most severe cases of the disease. Despite this, there was pressure to keep Nightingale open. However, knowing when and how to intervene intelligently using data and networks as opposed to emotion or the media were crucially important in influencing the next steps. The field of oncology is probably the fastest moving of any sphere of medicine and nursing—the entire landscape of treatment modalities is changing at breakneck speed. Oncology clinicians need to be politically aware; they need to know how to use data and outcomes to the benefit of our patients and our staff. As well as this, oncology professionals need to know who and how to access decision makers—whether this be healthcare leaders, research, political or media influencers.

Test Your Learning

1. What leadership models were used in this endeavour and how did they change over time?
2. Why were oncology professionals so prolific across leadership and care giving staff at the Nightingale?
3. What three things did you take from this chapter that you may bring back to your workplace tomorrow?

Post-script: Clearing the Garage

As I prepared to leave the Nightingale site that last Friday in May 2020, something caught my eye—it looked like a pile of rubbish by the bins. Curiosity got the better of me, and I wandered over to take a look. There, beside the garbage were piles and piles of Nightingale signage, protocols, maps, unused bedside documentation, blank staff certificates and even scores of the earliest architectural drawings and plans for the Nightingale; all were destined for the rubbish tip. I instinctively felt this *material* was important, and it just couldn't be destroyed. I filled my estate car to the brim with as much of this as I could safely fit, bearing in mind I had a 60-mile road trip to get home.

The contents of my car were decanted into my garage at home—Nightingale paraphernalia filled it from top to bottom. I then discussed the contents with colleagues, specifically, that I didn't know what to do with it.

A year passed and in late summer of 2021, I had a call from the 'Keeper of Medicine' at the Science Museum London. Word had spread regarding what I had salvaged. Could she take a team down to look at what I had rescued?

At this stage my mental health was frayed. I began to get anxious going into the garage—I couldn't look at any of the documents. I was struggling and wanted it all gone.

I carefully placed all of the documents and posters out; they covered my entire kitchen and dining room. The team from the Science Museum came and were overwhelmed. It was emotional as I told the story of each of the (now apparent) precious documents. The team said that as many were of national importance that they simply couldn't take them now and they would have to get a specialist team down to archive and remove them. I said take them all now or they are going in the bin—harsh, but I couldn't cope with them in my house for another day, and they needed to go to a special home. And with that they were gone.

My memories were not gone, as they are not from many staff, relatives and patients affected by the pandemic. I didn't know it at that time, but I was suffering with long Covid and later diagnosed with post-traumatic stress disorder (PTSD) as a result of my military and pandemic experiences. I got the help I needed from the NHS and have recovered, but I am also aware that many people have not recovered and the opening of the public enquiry into the pandemic in the United Kingdom will be a difficult time for many and my advice is for readers who may be triggered by this chapter to seek support from your line manager, occupational health department or general practitioner.

In the summer of 2022, we held a major healthcare conference at my hospital *'Looking Back but Moving Forward'* was the title—the day was based upon respecting and never forgetting those difficult days, but also moving forward with the learning and exemplary teamwork of those times.

Conflict of Interest The author has no conflict of interest to declare.

Open Access This chapter is licensed under the terms of the Creative Commons Attribution 4.0 International License (http://creativecommons.org/licenses/by/4.0/), which permits use, sharing, adaptation, distribution and reproduction in any medium or format, as long as you give appropriate credit to the original author(s) and the source, provide a link to the Creative Commons license and indicate if changes were made.

The images or other third party material in this chapter are included in the chapter's Creative Commons license, unless indicated otherwise in a credit line to the material. If material is not included in the chapter's Creative Commons license and your intended use is not permitted by statutory regulation or exceeds the permitted use, you will need to obtain permission directly from the copyright holder.

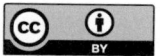

Cancer Patient Management and Flow During the COVID-19 Pandemic

11

Mark Foulkes

Check Your Experience
1. What changes to cancer pathways did you notice in your practice that resulted in a profound impact on patient care in terms of diagnosis, treatment and support needs as a consequence of the COVID-19 pandemic?
2. Of the adaptations made to cancer pathways in response to the COVID-19 pandemic, are there any which you feel should be maintained as they represent improvements in patient care and outcomes?

Introduction

As with all aspects of healthcare delivery, the COVID-19 pandemic has had a seismic effect on the manner in which patients with a suspected or confirmed diagnosis of cancer were managed and treated across the United Kingdom and Europe.

In the first months of the pandemic, all countries experienced a substantial drop in patients referred to hospitals with suspected cancer and hence in numbers subsequently diagnosed. In England, there were around 3500 fewer people diagnosed with cancer between April and August 2020 than might have been predicted from data derived from previous years [1].

This picture of a very significant decline in the number of patients diagnosed with cancer was seen across Europe [2, 3]. In late 2020 the European Cancer Organisation summarised the effects of COVID-19 pandemic on cancer pathways as:

- A stalling of cancer prevention programmes (such as HPV vaccination).
- A suspension of cancer screening and early detection programmes.

M. Foulkes (✉)
Macmillan Lead Cancer Nurse and Nurse Consultant,
Royal Berkshire NHS Foundation Trust, Reading, UK
e-mail: mark.foulkes@royalberkshire.nhs.uk

© The Author(s) 2026
M. Foulkes et al. (eds.), *Cancer Care in the Post-COVID World*,
https://doi.org/10.1007/978-3-031-33855-7_11

- The emergency situation across healthcare in 2020 deterred people with potential cancer symptoms from seeking medical advice.
- Delays in delivering all modalities of cancer treatment to varying degrees of severity and impaired follow-up to patients already treated.
- Clinical trials and the development of new agents and techniques negatively affected.
- A widening of inequalities in accessing cancer treatments.

These effects have resulted in an increased number of patients presenting with more advanced cancer and requiring assessment and treatment. Many health systems are struggling to cope. A commission from the Lancet Oncology brought together a range of patients alongside scientific and healthcare experts, all with knowledge of cancer across Europe. The report estimated that around one million cancer diagnoses were missed in Europe during the pandemic and postulated that many of these would have still undiagnosed cancer [4]. The sequelae of the pandemic were felt acutely across Europe and defined how health services approach cancer care and policy.

Screening Services and COVID-19

Cancer screening services internationally showed a profound decline in patient numbers during 2020 in the months directly following the declaration of the pandemic. Allahqoli et al. [5] reviewed 481 papers relating to screening programmes from across the world and found reductions in numbers in European countries for breast, cervical and colon cancer screening varied from 40% to 90% of pre-COVID levels of activity. The authors attributed these reductions to patients' fear of infection, stay-at-home orders, the redeployment of staff towards critical care for the management of COVID-19 patients and logistical issues relating to managing potential infection in patients attending for procedures. They also found that estimations of excess cancer mortality relating to screening disruption were likely to be in the order of 20% with most excess deaths probably occurring before 2025.

If we consider specific screening programmes, we find that the overall picture of significant reductions and loss of patient confidence is corroborated.

In mammogram-based breast screening, the picture of massive reductions of screening services during 2020 can be illustrated by the experience of the Netherlands, with a 60% reduction continuing until June of that year and a 40% reduction continuing until around September [6]. In Hungary, Elek et al. [7] found that it was likely many patients remained undiagnosed during the pandemic and that lower rates of partial mastectomies during and following the pandemic implied that some patients could have been diagnosed at an earlier stage with screening. A systemic review on the effects of the COVID-19 pandemic on breast screening found that there was evidence of more women presenting with higher-stage disease during and immediately after the declaration of the pandemic. There was little evidence of longer-term effects on the staging of breast cancer [8].

Carcopino et al. [9] found that cervical screening programmes across 31 European countries were suspended during 2020 and by December 2020 only 57% of countries had managed to recommence their programmes. The authors anticipated significant increases in the incidence of cervical cancer in the immediate post-pandemic years.

Colorectal screening programmes employ both invasive methods (colonoscopy, flexible sigmoidoscopy and CT colonography) and non-invasive methods such as faecal immunochemical test (FIT) and guaiac-based faecal occult blood test (gFOBT). Within these screening programmes, researchers conducted a systematic literature review of international literature and found very significant reductions in invasive screening procedures. An accompanying drop in non-invasive screening was first resolved and then showed higher levels of usage. The same research postulated that, worldwide, delays in diagnosis due to the COVID-19 epidemic were likely to cause a significant increase in the number of preventable colorectal cancer deaths, but this could be countered by a range of practical measures. These included replacing invasive screening with non-invasive methods and increasing capacity within screening centres post-restriction to compensate for the reduction during the time of restrictions [10].

In summary, the COVID-19 pandemic radically reduced the effectiveness of cancer screening programmes; particularly whilst restrictions were in place, the situation was further compounded by some programmes being slow to recover. This reduced effectiveness resulted in increases in the number of cancer diagnoses and/or an increase in diagnoses of cancer at a more advanced stage than pre-pandemic in those tumour sites where screening is a well-established means of detecting cancers.

Referral Pathway Effects

There are a range of routes by which people who have signs or symptoms of cancer may be referred for investigation and diagnosis. The main, and largely preferred, methodology is for the individual with symptoms to report these symptoms initially to their general practitioner (community doctor) or dentist. Research has indicated that this is largely effective and results in a better patient experience of the process of the diagnostic phase than those who arrive via other routes [11]. Many nations attempt to make this route as time-bounded and effective as possible. Patients may also be referred by their community doctor without clear suspicion of cancer for non-specific medical issues such as anaemia, back pain or weight loss. Cancer may then be detected whilst the referred patient is having investigations. These routine referrals are an important route via which cancer diagnoses can be made with analysis from the United Kingdom revealing that only around half of patients are diagnosed via a rapid cancer referral [12].

Other main referral routes include via screening services described above or via emergency presentation. Emergency presentations occur when a patient attends hospital due to an onset of acute symptoms which cannot be managed by the individual in the community. Examples of this would be when a patient presented in the emergency department with pain, severe bleeding, vomiting, confusion or falls. Outside of the COVID-19 pandemic, continuous research and audit from the United Kingdom would indicate that patients who present as an emergency tend to have worse outcomes than those who are referred in a more controlled manner across all tumour sites [13].

During the restrictions imposed by governments during the pandemic in mid-2020, referrals from community doctors in primary care reduced drastically as did non-COVID attendances at emergency departments. It seems likely that during this period people simply stopped reporting cancer symptoms via any route. However, later in 2020 from the United Kingdom, there is evidence that in some tumour sites, this period of non-reporting then led to an increase in people presenting via emergency departments with more advanced cancers. This evidence exists in head and neck cancers [14, 15] and in lung cancer, with increases in the number of emergency presentations with lung cancer [16] and lung cancers presenting at a more advanced stage [17]. Also, considering data (July–December 2020) from the United Kingdom, despite the total number of emergency presentations of cancer being below the pre-COVID levels, these represented a higher proportion of cancer diagnoses than pre-COVID pandemic [18].

The collapse in referrals to hospitals from community doctors in the United Kingdom can be seen in the graph below (see Fig. 11.1), illustrating the differences in urgent cancer referrals between 2020 and 2019. Most, but not all, tumour sites recovered to pre-COVID levels by early 2021 in the United Kingdom. By late 2021

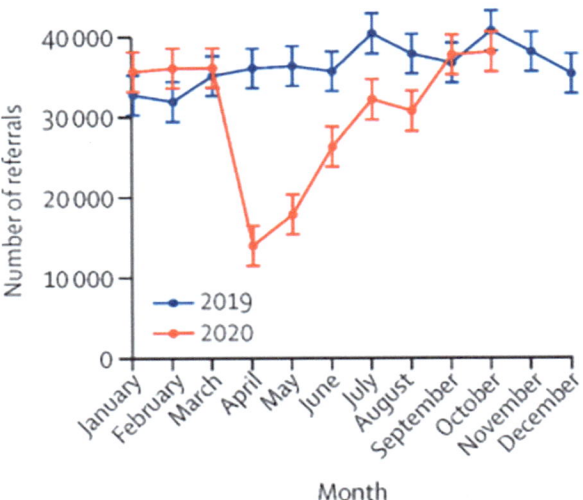

Fig. 11.1 Graph showing the United Kingdom monthly number of referrals into the urgent cancer pathway [20]

the referral numbers exceeded those seen before the pandemic, perhaps representing a proportion of patients who had not presented during this period.

In late 2020 and into early 2021 in the United Kingdom, the major challenge was restoring patient confidence in cancer services. Concerns about contracting COVID-19 became intertwined with pressure to reduce the demand on health services. Individuals in health systems realised that prolonged periods where patients did not present with cancer symptoms would result in a health crisis. Strategies were then set in motion to encourage patients to contact their community doctors with cancer symptoms and be referred in 'as usual'. Other strategies were put in place to deliver cancer treatments safely and reassure the public of their safety in hospital environments.

As fears of contracting SARS-CoV-2 in the general population have reduced, and with the emergence of effective vaccination, the major issue in most cancer services shifted from encouraging patients to attend hospital to dealing with increased demand for cancer care from a COVID backlog and aging populations.

Effects on Diagnostics

Once a patient is referred to a hospital, the detection of a cancer relies upon the effective use of diagnostic tests. These can be radiological in nature, such as X-rays and scans, or more invasive, such as endoscopy or biopsy. From March 2020 when the COVID pandemic was declared, there was a significant reduction in diagnostic tests being performed across Europe. In the United Kingdom between March and August, 35% fewer diagnostic tests were performed compared to the same period in 2019 [19]. Inevitably fewer diagnostic tests lead to fewer actual diagnoses, and as a result, reduced cancer diagnoses were noted across Europe [4].

More invasive tests, particularly endoscopic procedures, were negatively affected. As an example, in England there was a 92% reduction in the number of colonoscopies performed during April 2020 compared with during the same month in 2019 [20] Rutter et al. [21] outline the process whereby, in the United Kingdom, nearly all endoscopic procedures were stopped in the early days of the pandemic. This was due to concerns around upper gastrointestinal endoscopy (such as gastroscopy) being a high-risk 'aerosol-generating procedure' (AGP) and lower GI endoscopy subjecting staff to shedding of the SARS-CoV-2 virus from faeces. They also describe the slow recovery of endoscopic services in the United Kingdom attributing this to staff shortages (due to redeployment, illness and shielding/self-isolation) as well as the restructuring of endoscopic services, the need for social distancing, greatly increased cleaning between procedures and personal protective equipment (PPE) application and removal, all of which dramatically reduced patient throughput. By the end of May 2020, endoscopic procedures were still only 20% of pre-COVID levels.

By the end of 2020 and into 2021, endoscopy units were beginning to build significant backlogs of patients awaiting procedures. During this time period, organisations that worked together to pool endoscopic resources and provide 'mutual aid' for each other were more successful at reducing waiting times and backlogs. This pooling of resources allowed for the movement of lists between units and the free movement of endoscopy staff to units where they were needed [22].

The significant impact of the pandemic on diagnostic endoscopy has resulted in real learning which should be used to make services more resilient in the face of other major systemic challenges. These changes will include the adoption and maintenance of effective levels of PPE, well-managed and segregated recovery areas, improved training (some of which can be provided 'virtually') and a more effective management of delayed or abandoned procedures [23]. An interesting innovation has been the further development of non-endoscopic form of gastrointestinal tract imaging such as 'capsule endoscopy' whereby a small camera is swallowed, and images are transmitted to a recording device worn or carried by the patient. There is increasing evidence that, in some cases, this could be an effective alternative to invasive endoscopy [24].

As with most hospital-based procedures, radiology departments delivering X-rays, CT, MRI and PET scanning were initially hit very hard by the first weeks of the COVID-19 pandemic. The evidence is, however, that in most European nations, radiological imaging was able to recover relatively quickly in comparison to more invasive diagnostic procedures. It became apparent that functional radiological services could be established safely in the presence of the SARS-CoV-2 virus should patients wish to access them and the logistics be in place to do this. Research from Italy, examining the reasons why more lung cancers presented at a more advanced stage than pre-pandemic, identified that a lack of willingness to present to health services with symptoms was the most likely cause rather than diagnostic delays [25]. Services delivered by UK diagnostic radiology departments were remodelled to facilitate care for both COVID-19 and non-COVID patients, whilst they struggled to meet unprecedented demand for medical imaging to confirm COVID-19 diagnosis and extent of disease. As with many staff groups working through the pandemic, it was clear that the diagnostic radiology workforce suffered considerable stress during this period and many personal and service-based challenges [26]. The two factors driving this have been cited as:

- Implementation of personal protective equipment (PPE) and changes to infection-control guidelines.
- Extensive changes to normal processes and practices such as increased working hours, restructuring of workforce and resources and changes to well-established departmental protocols.

Effects on Treatment

Managing Staff and Workforce Strategies

In the immediate aftermath of the international declaration of the pandemic, with Europe being the epicentre, the rate of sickness around 20% was commonplace amongst health workers. This was not only because of personal sickness through contracting the SARS-CoV-2 virus but also due to self-isolating due to symptoms of infection, or because of COVID-19 infection, or symptoms of the same, being present in family members. The impact of this level of sickness would have been much more significant if it had not been mediated by a fall in the number of treatments delivered due to adaptation, deferral or moves to non-face-to-face appointments [27].

Following lessons from previous pandemics in South East Asia, separating health provision between COVID- and non-COVID-infected areas became commonplace in order to reduce the risk of nosocomial infection. Due to the perceived risk of SARS-CoV-2 virus infection affecting immunosuppressed patients in cancer care, moving oncology away from acute areas was the logical extension of this. In 2020, in the United Kingdom, the relocation of cancer teams and services away from general hospitals caring for patients with COVID-19 was a commonly employed strategy. The underpinning idea was to form centralised 'hubs' for cancer treatment and cancer surgery, so that patients did not need to attend hospitals with a high risk of encountering the virus. Consolidating cancer treatment in cancer hubs kept as free as possible from SARS-CoV-2 exposure in the United Kingdom echoed a similar policy in the North of Italy [28]. These models recommended geographically distinct cancer-care facilities from those treating COVID-19. This was not always possible, and separate facilities were employed on mixed-care sites with services delivered by a specific, and tested, pool of staff. This reduced the risk of exposing COVID-free patients and healthcare workers to the virus [29]. It is not possible to determine the effectiveness of these strategies on overall morbidity and mortality for patients diagnosed with cancer during the COVID-19 pandemic. The widespread relocation of cancer services and the consequent redeployment of oncology staff had a negative impact on the recovery of services both in terms of logistics and the well-being and mental health of oncology healthcare workers, which is discussed in more detail in Chap. 9.

In addition, the pandemic amplified pre-existing shortfalls in healthcare workers specialising in oncology; these would include cross-Europe shortages of oncologists, radiographers and cancer nurses. This impact was felt particularly within cancer nursing. Cancer nurses have specific skills in communicating in challenging situations, and in infection control, and because of this, during each wave of the pandemic, they were pulled from their regular duties to COVID-19 wards or other intensive areas [30]. With the advent of effective vaccination and improved access to testing of oncology professionals, the workforce stabilised, but the COVID-19 pandemic exacerbated existing issues such as an aging workforce and low number of oncologists, nurses and radiographers in training, and economies across Europe continue to struggle to meet the challenge of increasing demand on cancer services.

With effective vaccination, there was the additional issue of how to manage staff who did not wish to be vaccinated. In the United Kingdom, vaccination for patient-facing staff was made mandatory, with some staff facing dismissal if they declined vaccination. This decision was then reversed in early 2022 with the realisation this would exacerbate workforce shortages.

Surgery

For many types of cancer, surgical removal remains the gold-standard treatment and is frequently employed in combination with non-surgical modalities such as radiotherapy and delivery of systemic anti-cancer treatments (SACT). Intubation of surgical patients constitutes a high-risk aerosol-generating procedure (AGP), and people who develop COVID-19 around the time of their surgery are more likely than people without the infection to have complications and to die [31]. In addition, in the first days of the COVID pandemic, staff working in a theatre carried a high risk of infection with the SARS-CoV-2 virus [32]. This was particularly true of surgeons and other healthcare workers working in the field of Ear, Nose and Throat who carried a significantly higher risk of exposure to the SARS-CoV-2 virus, infection and hospitalisation [33]. It therefore became imperative that this risk was managed in order to maintain the surgical management of patients with cancer and other diseases which required urgent and life-saving surgery. The methodologies employed across Europe to deliver surgical management can be separated into three main groups, logistical, testing, and prioritisation/risk assessment.

1. Logistics: As described previously, many healthcare organisations developed an approach which separated surgical patients from the general hospital population in order to reduce the risk of nosocomial infection. This was either done by the creation of centralised, regional surgical 'hubs' taking patients from a number of different hospitals, or, where this was not possible, creating secure surgical pathways within hospitals. Effective and successful examples of this methodology were seen in London (UK) [34] and in Italy [35]. This approach required patients to travel for surgery, to be tested prior to admission and for there to be a secure methodology for keeping patients and surgical staff separate from the general population. Although, on the face of it, the creation of surgical hubs seemed disruptive to individual services and pathways, data from the United Kingdom particularly suggests that this technique was effective and reduced surgical morbidity [34].
2. Testing: As effective testing became more widely available, it became apparent that this was vital in order to keep surgical pathways safe and prevent operations being carried out on patients with SARS-CoV-2 infection. Patients were, required to complete polymerase chain testing (PCR) and/or rapid lateral flow (LFT) testing prior to admission as well as screening questionnaires. This was rapidly added to guidelines and protocols in most European nations [36]. A major issue around testing was to ensure that testing was carried out at an appropriate point

prior to surgery to reduce the chance of SARS-CoV-2 exposure and infection between testing and surgery taking place. In many cases patients were required to be tested and then self-isolate for a number of days prior to admission [37]. This led to a number of logistical issues in ensuring compliance and managing this process.

In addition to non-symptomatic patient testing, staff testing became routine, although, across Europe, there were considerable, and variable, delays in offering this due to the availability and accessibility of testing. In the United Kingdom, guidance was published in June 2020 recommending healthcare workers in regular contact with patients on non-surgical oncology pathways should be routinely tested, even if asymptomatic [38]. From limited evidence available, it seems surgical pathways did not adopt this advice until later in 2020. Pan-Europe guidance outlining the need for routine testing of asymptomatic health workers was not published until September 2020 [39], with the same document highlighting the variation in practice across European nations.

3. Surgical prioritisation: As we have seen above, in the first year of the pandemic in Europe, surgical capacity was severely challenged, and attempts were made to prioritise groups of non-COVID-infected patients needing surgical intervention. In the United Kingdom, this was formulated around the time that could elapse before the individual's outcome would be seriously compromised and was derived from the Royal College of Surgeons of England advice [40].
Priority level 1a (emergency)—operation needed within 24 h to save life.
Priority level 1b (urgent)—operation needed within 72 h.
Priority level 2—elective surgery with the expectation of cure, prioritised within 4 weeks to save life/progression of disease beyond operability.
Priority level 3—elective surgery delayed for 10–12 weeks will have no predicted negative outcome.

The expectation was that all complex cancer surgery would require level 1 support routinely. This prioritisation scheme allowed for the management of resources and collaboration to ensure high-priority cases were operated on within the advised timescale.

Systemic Anti-cancer Therapy (SACT) Delivery

At the beginning of the pandemic, most European nations were cautious about continuing to routinely deliver SACT, as the effect of SARS-CoV-2 infection on patients who were immunosuppressed was unclear. There was some evidence from China that this group was at higher risk of contracting the virus and with worse outcomes if this did occur [41]. This uncertainty led to a sudden drop in the delivery of SACT in the first 4–6 weeks of the pandemic, with, for example, a 28% drop in Scotland [42], a 45–66% drop in England and Northern Ireland [43] and a 31% drop in the

Netherlands [44]. In response to this anxiety, most European nations produced guidance around the delivery of SACT, which frequently suggested risk-stratifying treatment regimens by their likely impact on immunosuppression, the risk of success of the regimen and the risks associated with contracting SARS-CoV-2 [45]. This inevitably led to many difficult conversations with patients who experienced SACT regimens not commencing, being changed, or even being suspended. In addition to this, guidelines largely recommended that patients receiving SACT should self-isolate as much as possible and reduce social contacts. As testing became more widely available, the emphasis shifted to patient and staff testing. Largely, the advice to self-isolate or 'shield' continued throughout the pandemic and even after. As with most areas of cancer care, these pathway changes led to many logistical challenges in delivering SACT and lessons learned for staff working in these areas.

Radiotherapy

As with diagnostic radiography, therapeutic radiography was initially affected widely during the first weeks of the pandemic, but services were able to adapt reasonably quickly [26]. Research from the United Kingdom would suggest that there was an overall drop in the fractions of radiotherapy delivered during 2020/2021, but this drop was less marked than in surgery or SACT delivery [46].

The clinical effectiveness of changes to radiotherapy practice was tested rapidly in radiotherapy departments as an international consensus statement was reached recommending short-course radiotherapy for rectal cancers as a means of delaying surgical excision [47]. In the field of breast cancer, the timely publication of the 'FAST-Forward' trial results [48] enabled the duration of radiotherapy treatment to be shortened. For other groups of patients, such as those with prostate cancer, radiotherapy for localised disease was deferred in order to build capacity for referrals resulting from reductions in surgery and the initially cautious approach to delivering SACT.

Within the field of oncology, it appeared that radiotherapy services were some of the first to treat patients with a known positive COVID-19 status, and, as with diagnostic radiography services, this led to high levels of COVID-related sickness, anxiety and concerns around personal protective equipment and infection control protocols [26].

Oncology Follow-Up

Most patients who experience a cancer diagnosis require monitoring pre-, during and post-treatments. In some cases, patients with advanced disease may not be receiving active oncological interventions; however, they still require monitoring and care. Prior to the COVID-19 pandemic, this monitoring and care would be achieved via a multiprofessional approach with a mixture of hospital attendance for regular appointments, community care, structured patient-initiated follow-up (PIFU) (largely via secondary care) and specialist services such as palliative care.

There is a wide range of evidence that this network of care was drastically disrupted by the COVID-19 pandemic. Research carried out by Cancer Research UK in the UK indicated that around 64% of patients experienced a deterioration in the standard of their care with individuals reporting feelings of abandonment, particularly by their oncology teams within hospitals but also in terms of community services such as support groups [49]. Research from Germany indicated that of the patients who felt their care had been affected by the pandemic, 72% reported a change in follow-up care arrangements [50].

Whilst disruption to screening, diagnostic services and treatment has direct effects on the survivability of a cancer diagnosis, shortfalls and major changes to the way people with cancer are cared for and supported post-treatment have the potential to negatively impact their mental health and general well-being. The changes patients were most likely to experience during the pandemic in their follow-up and support services were a move from face-to-face to telephone and video consultations and reduced access to their own oncology teams (medical and other healthcare professionals) [50, 51]. In the post-pandemic era, patients are able to access their own oncology teams with greater ease, but longer-term changes have been made to the way patients are followed up, with a greater emphasis on non-face-to-face appointments and a greater use of technology. As you will read elsewhere in this publication, there are both positive aspects to this and some areas which are yet to be proven in terms of patient benefit (see Chapters [4, 5]).

Although possible changes regarding follow-up arrangements were being explored and developed prior to the COVID-19 pandemic, some authors have indicated that an extension of patient-initiated follow-up (PIFU) schemes in cancer care might address some of the challenges thrown up by the pandemic [50]. PIFU schemes (also known as supported early discharge, open access or stratified follow-up) aim to empower patients to manage their own condition by taking responsibility for initiating appointments themselves when they note symptoms of concern. In cancer care such schemes would also include an element of holistic assessment, care planning and a high level of information support prior to accessing the scheme if they are to meet patient needs [52]. They typically reduce the need for patients to attend structured clinic appointments in secondary care but do require skilled, high-quality interventions, from a highly skilled professional, usually specialist nurses, before patients are discharged onto a PIFU scheme. It does not appear that PIFU was increased widely in the United Kingdom during the pandemic, but the move towards extending PIFU, certainly in the United Kingdom, is gathering pace.

Long-Term Impacts on Cancer Pathways

As we have seen in this chapter, there is no doubt that the pandemic had a substantial and sustained disruptive effect on cancer services across Europe during the first two years post March 2020. Modelling indicates that the missed opportunities to screen patients and to offer timely treatment due to this disruption will result in increased numbers of patients presenting with more advanced cancers until around

2030 [53]. It is therefore likely that these increased presentations will put additional pressure on already stretched resources in healthcare.

Other longer-term effects are more difficult to quantify, but cancer services have developed increased resilience, particularly to major disruptions caused by a pandemic. The pace of learning and the rapid responses to challenges have taught clinicians and managers that it is possible to maintain services in the most difficult circumstances and that effective, timely decision-making is possible and desirable in a crisis. It is yet to be seen how many of the rapid changes to pathways instigated by the pandemic will be maintained longer term as they are seen as positive or desirable.

Some authors have postulated that the COVID infection, as with other viruses, may precipitate increased cancer incidence. The effects of the unique types of inflammatory cascades associated with COVID-19 alongside the excessive inflammation, alteration of cellular signalling pathways and exhaustion of immune function may cause cancers to arise or dormant cancer cells to become active [54]. These effects are currently largely theoretical, and it remains to be seen if these occur in nature over time.

It may be that the biggest impact of a cancer diagnosis, treatments and follow-up has been the loss of public confidence in how individuals with cancer can be kept safe whilst moving through cancer pathways. It is difficult to assess how long this effect will be felt and what is the most effective manner to address it.

Test Your Learning

What evidence is there that disruption of screening programmes across Europe and the United Kingdom resulted in a negative impact on the effectiveness of cancer pathways?

As healthcare professionals, what have we learned from the impact of the pandemic on cancer pathways in your area of practice?

What would we change in the way systems should respond to future pandemics, and why?

References

1. Morris E, Goldacre R et al (2021) Impact of the COVID-19 pandemic on the detection and management of colorectal cancer in England: a population-based study. Lancet Gastroenterol Hepatol 6:199–208
2. Johansson ALV, Laronningen S et al (2022) The impact of the COVID-19 pandemic on cancer diagnosis based on pathology notifications: a comparison across the Nordic countries during 2020. Int J Cancer 151(3):381–395
3. Dinmohamed AG, Visser O et al (2020) Fewer cancer diagnoses during the Covid-19 epidemic in the Netherlands. Lancet Oncol 21:750–751
4. Lawler M, Davies L et al (2022) European Groundshot – addressing Europe's cancer research challenges: a Lancet Oncology Commission. Published on-line November 15. https://doi.org/10.1016/S1470-2045(22)00540-X
5. Allahqoli L, Mazidimoradi A, Salehiniya H, Alkatout I (2022) Impact of COVID-19 on cancer screening: a global perspective. Curr Opin Support Palliat Care 16(3):102–109

6. Eijkelboom AH, De Munck L, Lobbeset M (2021) Impact of the suspension and restart of the Dutch breast cancer screening program on breast cancer incidence and stage during the COVID-19 pandemic. Prev Med 151:106602
7. Elek P, Fadgyas-Freyler P, Varadi B, Mayer B, Zemplenyi A, Csanadi M (2022) Effects of lower screening activity during the COVID-19 pandemic on breast cancer patient pathways: evidence from the age cut-off of organized screening. Health Policy 126:763–769
8. Li T et al (2023) A systematic review of the impact of the COVID-19 pandemic on breast cancer screening and diagnosis. Breast 67:78–88
9. Carcopino X, Cruickshank M, Leeson S, Redman C, Nieminen P (2022) The impact of COVID-19 pandemic on screening programs for cervical cancer prevention across Europe. J Lower Genital Tract Dis 26(3):219–222
10. Mazidimoradi A, Tiznobaik A, Salehiniya H (2022) Impact of the COVID-19 pandemic on colorectal cancer screening: a systematic review. J Gastrointest Cancer 53(3):730–744
11. Sandager M, Jensen H, Lipczak H, Sperling CD, Vedsted P (2019) 'Cancer patients' experiences with urgent referrals to cancer patient pathways. Eur J Cancer Care 28(1):e12927
12. Zhou Y et al (2017) Variation in 'fast-track' referrals for suspected cancer by patient characteristic and cancer diagnosis: evidence from 670000 patients with cancers of 35 different sites. Br J Cancer 118:24–31
13. Ellis-Brooks L (2018) Routes to diagnosis – driving improvements in cancer with a decade of data. UK Health Security Agency Blog. https://ukhsa.blog.gov.uk/2018/01/17/routes-to-diagnosis-driving-improvements-in-cancer-with-a-decade-of-data/. Last accessed January 2023
14. Stringer H, Mohammed N, Mumtaz S, Komath D (2022) Head and neck cancer presentations in the emergency department during the COVID-19 pandemic. Br Dent J. Online Publication
15. Metzger K, Mrosek J, Zittel S et al (2021) Treatment delay and tumour size in patients with oral cancer during the first year of the COVID-19 pandemic. Head Neck 43:3493–3497
16. Vella C, Ashraf A, Sudhir R et al (2021) Increase in lung cancer emergency presentations during the COVID-19 pandemic. Eur Respir J 58(Suppl 65):PA3848
17. Ramos Pereira A, Coombs C, Masterman B, Jeyabalan A, Plummeridge M, Bibby A (2022) Impact of the COVID-19 pandemic on suspected lung cancer referrals and subsequent lung cancer diagnosis at North Bristol NHS Trust. Eur Respir J 60(Suppl 66):139
18. Public Health England (2021) Emergency presentations of cancer: data up to December 2020. https://www.gov.uk/government/statistics/emergency-presentations-of-cancer-data-up-to-december-2020/emergency-presentations-of-cancer-data-up-to-december-2020. Last accessed March 2023
19. Greenwood E, Swanton C (2021) Consequences of COVID-19 for cancer care – a CRUK perspective. Nat Rev Clin Oncol 18:3–4
20. Morris EJA, Goldacre R, Spata E, Mafham M, Finan PJ, Shelton J, Richards M, Spencer K, Emberson J, Hollings S et al (2021) Impact of the COVID-19 pandemic on the detection and management of colorectal cancer in England: a population-based study. Lancet Gastroenterol Hepatol 6:199–208
21. Rutter MD, Brookes M, Lee TJ et al (2021) Impact of the COVID-19 pandemic on UK endoscopic activity and cancer detection: a national endoscopy database analysis. Gut 70:537–543
22. NHS Confederation (2021) Recovering endoscopy services during the COVID-19 pandemic. https://www.nhsconfed.org/case-studies/recovering-endoscopy-services-during-covid-19-pandemic. Last accessed January 2023
23. Lui RN, Tang RSY, Chiu PWY (2022) Endoscopy after the COVID-19 Pandemic – what will be different? Curr Treat Options Gastroenterol 20:46–59
24. Koulaouzidis G, Robertson A, Wenzek H et al (2022) Colon capsule endoscopy: the evidence is piling up. Gut 71:440–441
25. Cantini L, Mentrasti G, Russo GL et al (2022) Evaluation of COVID-19 impact on DELAYing diagnostic-therapeutic pathways of lung cancer patients in Italy (COVID-DELAY study): fewer cases and higher stages from a real-world scenario. ESMO Open 7(2):100406

26. McFadden S, Flood T, Shepherd P, Gilleece T (2022) Impact of COVID-19 on service delivery in radiology and radiotherapy. Radiography 28(Supp 1):S16–S26
27. Mayor S (2020) COVID-19: impact on cancer workforce and delivery of care. Lancet Oncol 21(5):633
28. Curigliano G (2020) The treatment of patients with cancer and containment of COVID-19: experiences from Italy. ASCO Daily News, March 17, 2020. https://dailynews.ascopubs.org/do/treatment-patients-cancer-and-containment-covid-19-experiences-italy. Last accessed January 2023
29. Richards M, Anderson M, Carter P et al (2020) The impact of the COVID-19 pandemic on cancer care. Nat Cancer 1:565–567
30. Woodford E (2022) How to tackle the COVID-19 curve-ball in cancer care. European Policy Centre, Policy Brief: Social Europe & Well-Being Programme. https://www.epc.eu/content/publications/C19_and_Cancer_care_PB_v3.pdf. Last accessed January 2023
31. COVIDSurg Collaborative (2021) Machine learning risk prediction of mortality for patients undergoing surgery with perioperative SARS-CoV-2: the COVIDSurg mortality score. Br J Surg 108(11):1274–1292
32. Hou J et al (2020) COVID-19 infection, a potential threat to surgical patients and staff? A retrospective cohort study. Int J Surg 82:172–178
33. Couloigner V et al (2020) COVID-19 and ENT surgery. Eur Ann Otorhinolaryngol Head Neck Dis 137(3):161–166
34. Kayani B, Roberts L, Haddad FS (2020) Developing a surgical oncology hub during the COVID-19 pandemic: lessons learned from the United Kingdom. J Br Surg 107(11):e510–e511
35. Sorrentino L, Guaglio M, Cosimelli M (2020) Elective colorectal cancer surgery at the oncologic hub of Lombardy inside a pandemic COVID-19 area. J Surg Oncol 122(10):1002
36. Vecchione L et al (2020) ESMO management and treatment adapted recommendations in the COVID-19 era: colorectal cancer. ESMO Open 5. https://www.esmo.org/guidelines/cancer-patient-management-during-the-covid-19-pandemic. Last accessed January 2023
37. Discombe M (2020) Patients must isolate for two weeks before an NHS operation. Health Serv J. https://www.hsj.co.uk/coronavirus/patients-must-isolate-for-two-weeks-before-an-nhs-operation/7027653.article. Last accessed March 2023
38. Roques T, Board R (2020) Guidance on SARS-CoV-2 antigen testing for asymptomatic healthcare workers (HCW) and patients in non-surgical oncology in the UK. https://www.rcr.ac.uk/college/coronavirus-covid-19-what-rcr-doing/coronavirus-covid-19-clinical-oncology-resources. Last accessed January 2023
39. The European Commission Directorate-General for Health and Food Safety (2020) EU health preparedness: recommendations for a common EU testing approach for COVID-19. https://health.ec.europa.eu/system/files/2020-09/common_testingapproach_covid-19_en_0.pdf. Last accessed January 2023
40. NHS Speciality guides for patient management during the coronavirus pandemic (2020) Clinical guide for the management of non-coronavirus patients requiring acute treatment: cancer. Publications approval reference: 001559. https://www.nice.org.uk/Media/Default/About/COVID-19/Specialty-guides/cancer-and-COVID-19.pdf. Last accessed January 2023
41. Dai M, Liu D, Liu M, Zhou F, Li G, Chen Z et al (2020) Patients with cancer appear more vulnerable to SARS-COV-2: a multi-center study during the COVID-19 outbreak. Cancer Discov 10(6):83–791
42. Baxter MA, Murphy J, Cameron D et al (2021) The impact of COVID-19 on systemic anticancer treatment delivery in Scotland. Br J Cancer 124:1353–1356
43. Lai AG, Pasea L, Banerjee A, Hall G, Denaxas S, Chang WH et al (2020) Estimated impact of the COVID-19 pandemic on cancer services and excess 1-year mortality in people with cancer and multimorbidity: near real-time data on cancer care, cancer deaths and a population-based cohort study. BMJ Open 10:e043828
44. De Joode K et al (2020) Impact of the coronavirus disease 2019 pandemic on cancer treatment: the patients' perspective. Eur J Cancer:132–139

45. Petrova D, Perez-Gomes B et al (2020) Implications of the COVID-19 pandemic for cancer in Spain. Med Clín (Engl Ed) 55(6):263–266
46. Spencer K et al (2021) The impact of the COVID-19 pandemic on radiotherapy services in England, UK: a population-based study. Lancet Oncol 22(6):e239
47. Marijnen CAM, Peters FP, Rödel C, Bujko K, Haustermans K, Fokas E et al (2020) International expert consensus statement regarding radiotherapy treatment options for rectal cancer during the COVID-19 pandemic. Radiother Oncol 148:213–215
48. Brunt AM, Haviland JS, Wheatley DA, Sydenham MA, Alhasso A, Bloomfield DJ et al (2020) Hypofractionated breast radiotherapy for 1 week versus 3 weeks (FAST-Forward): 5-year efficacy and late normal tissue effects results from a multicentre, non-inferiority, randomised, phase 3 trial. Lancet 395(10237):1613–1626
49. Cancer Research UK (2020) Cancer research UK cancer patient experience survey 2020: the impact of COVID-19 on cancer patients in the UK. https://www.cancerresearchuk.org/sites/default/files/pes_covid_2020.pdf. Last accessed January 2023
50. Eckford RD et al (2021) The COVID-19 pandemic and cancer patients in Germany: impact on treatment, follow-up care and psychological burden. Front Public Health 9:788598
51. Levell NJ (2022) NHS outpatient secondary care: a time of challenges and opportunities. Future Healthc J 9(2):106–112
52. Taylor C, Cummings R, McGilly C (2013) Holistic needs assessment following colorectal cancer treatment. Gastrointest Nurs 10(9):42–49
53. Duffy SW, Seedat F, Kearins O et al (2022) The projected impact of the COVID-19 lockdown on breast cancer deaths in England due to the cessation of population screening: a national estimation. Br J Cancer 126:1355–1361
54. Du Plessis M et al (2022) Cancer and Covid-19: collectively catastrophic. Cytokine Growth Factor Rev 63:78–89

Open Access This chapter is licensed under the terms of the Creative Commons Attribution 4.0 International License (http://creativecommons.org/licenses/by/4.0/), which permits use, sharing, adaptation, distribution and reproduction in any medium or format, as long as you give appropriate credit to the original author(s) and the source, provide a link to the Creative Commons license and indicate if changes were made.

The images or other third party material in this chapter are included in the chapter's Creative Commons license, unless indicated otherwise in a credit line to the material. If material is not included in the chapter's Creative Commons license and your intended use is not permitted by statutory regulation or exceeds the permitted use, you will need to obtain permission directly from the copyright holder.

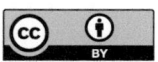

The Delivery of Systemic Anti-Cancer Therapies (SACT) During the COVID-19 Pandemic

12

Mark Foulkes

Check Your Knowledge and Experience
1. What were the main drivers in reducing the number of patients receiving SACT attending acute hospitals during the COVID-19 pandemic?
2. What do you believe were the negative effects of the reduction in planned attendances for patients receiving SACT?

Introduction

In the early days of the COVID-19 pandemic, there were major concerns that people with a cancer diagnosis were more prone to SARS-CoV-2 infection, and there was some evidence that they might also experience worse outcomes following infection than those in the general population [1]. There was little or no data which could be used to assess any additional effect of systemic anti-cancer therapy (SACT) on responses to SARS-CoV-2 infection. The immunosuppressive effects of cytotoxic chemotherapy were thought to add additional risk, but there were also unknown effects on the immune response to SARS-CoV-2 infection in individuals having treatment with more novel agents such as immune or targeted therapies. There was some speculation that the 'cytokine storm' associated with severe SARS-CoV-2 infection would adversely affect patients receiving checkpoint inhibitors.

Considering the evidence available at the time, both across Europe and the world, policies were put in place to try and protect patients receiving SACT from SARS-CoV-2 infection and to try and reduce the perceived risk of mortality and morbidity. Many of these measures were based on the principles of reducing treatments which increased risk for reduced benefit (such as patients receiving palliative treatments)

M. Foulkes (✉)
Macmillan Lead Cancer Nurse and Nurse Consultant,
Royal Berkshire NHS Foundation Trust, Reading, UK
e-mail: mark.foulkes@royalberkshire.nhs.uk

© The Author(s) 2026
M. Foulkes et al. (eds.), *Cancer Care in the Post-COVID World*,
https://doi.org/10.1007/978-3-031-33855-7_12

and reducing the risk of exposure to the SARS-CoV-2 virus (by reducing the number of visits to hospitals).

As the COVID-19 pandemic continued, more evidence began to emerge that the continued delivery of SACT did not significantly increase mortality in those patients continuing with treatment, perhaps with the notable exceptions of those patients with haematological malignancy and those from non-white ethnic backgrounds [2, 3].

As discussed in Chap. 11, the adjustments to the delivery of SACT had a considerable impact on cancer pathways with lower number of patients being treated with SACT across Europe and considerable patient distress where patients were reduced or curtailed. As we will see in this chapter, however, as the COVID-19 pandemic progressed and developed across Europe, particularly with the advent of effective vaccines, SACT delivery levels have returned to pre-pandemic levels and, in most cases, moved beyond these. There is no doubt that the pandemic period has had a negative effect on patients receiving SACT and those delivering it but also provided the impetus for innovations in SACT delivery, the benefits of which have extended beyond the COVID-19 pandemic and into routine clinical practice.

Adaptations to SACT Delivery in Response to the COVID-19 Pandemic

Closure and Relocation of SACT Units and Restriction of Visitors

In the early days of the COVID-19 pandemic, many SACT units were relocated away from main hospital sites with, in most cases, a total ban on patients having friends or relatives with them whilst receiving treatment. The thinking behind this was to protect immunosuppressed patients by providing safer routes in and out of the units and reducing the chances of staff transmission to patients. In addition, relocation allowed the repurposing of oncology units for caring for a high number of patients either with confirmed SARS-CoV-2 infection or those who had been exposed to the virus [4]. It is unclear how successful this was in protecting patients and the SACT workforce or simply a logistical process in order to free up capacity for the potentially high number of patients with SARS-CoV-2 infection. It is clear that this led to staff and patient isolation, pathway disruption and reduced capacity to treat patients. Whilst there is little evidence to support that moving SACT units away from acute hospitals and restricting visitors had any beneficial effects in reducing infection or promoting better clinical outcomes, there is clear evidence that the COVID-19 pandemic increased patient isolation and loneliness [5] with lack of visiting in chemotherapy and SACT units cited directly as a factor in the USA [6]. Here, a patient talks about her experience of receiving SACT at a centre in the United Kingdom during the COVID-19 pandemic, 'It was difficult to chat with other patients because we were socially distanced, which made it harder to make friends and it did feel quite isolating…..they (the nurses) were the only people I had interaction with throughout lockdown apart from my partner due to shielding'. [7]

Other major restrictions imposed by reduced visits to hospitals, specifically to SACT units, were patients' access to tests and processes which, although peripheral to the delivery of SACT, are vital in maintaining patient safety. An example of this would be the delivery of pretreatment systemic anti-cancer treatment (SACT) consultations. Before the COVID-19 pandemic, most cancer centres in the United Kingdom relied upon in-person assessments of patients prior to commencing SACT. These sessions were generally used to assess patients' knowledge, consider intravenous access, check consent and help familiarise patients with the SACT Unit. During COVID-19, these assessments were either stopped or curtailed making it more difficult to assess patients. Chap. 5 covers the effect of the COVID-19 pandemic on pre-assessment and some effective solutions to this.

The safe prescribing and administration of SACT rely upon the ability to assess patients' haematological response to anti-cancer agents. Most of these toxicities can be assessed via blood tests. Many of these take place in the community, and as access to community doctors was severely reduced, then these regular blood tests were very difficult to maintain. Data from the United Kingdom shows that in the first months of the pandemic (March to May 2020), tests carried out in primary (community) care dropped by 80%. By the end of June 2020, the number of tests being delivered was still less than half of the normal levels. [8] This reduction in community access meant that patients were more reliant on obtaining blood tests at hospitals where capacity was much challenged and the environment viewed as being higher risk for immunosuppressed patients. This reduced access to monitoring contributed to the changes made to some SACT regimens and the prioritisation of others discussed elsewhere (see Chap. 11) as well as to increased stress and concern for patients and families.

The Use of Online, 'Virtual' and Telephone SACT Assessments

As has been discussed widely elsewhere, and in detail in Chap. 5, the use of telemedicine in assessing patients receiving SACT expanded rapidly during the COVID-19 pandemic. Certainly during the pandemic itself and in the immediate post-pandemic period, most centres delivering SACT across Europe moved to a position where in-person attendances of patients with a cancer diagnosis were reduced to a minimum. From the available research, this move seems to have been largely well tolerated by patients, with no deterioration in patient experience or outcomes [9]. However, a recent scoping review of reviews in The Lancet [10] found that there were gaps in the literature with no studies specifically addressing older adults or the sustainability of interventions, and only two reviews focused on comparing telehealth to in-person interventions. In order to assess the long-term effectiveness of these interventions, these gaps would need to be addressed as well as a more thorough approach to gathering evidence relating to telehealth in SACT delivery.

Move to Oral and Sub-Cut Delivery and Self-Administration

As the COVID-19 pandemic first became established in the United Kingdom and Europe, a key early strategy in reducing the number of visits to a hospital and the time spent there was to maximise the doses of SACT that could be given via the oral or subcutaneous route.

The use of oral SACT agents has been well-established for many years, the main challenges of working in this way being ensuring that the patient and other healthcare workers know that the side effects and dangers of delivering oral SACT are exactly the same as receiving the intravenous (IV) versions of the agents. The patient therefore requires good levels of monitoring and patient and carer education as the delivery of the SACT is not generally witnessed or directly supervised by a healthcare professional. Examples of well-established oral agents are capecitabine in bowel and breast cancer and vinorelbine in breast and lung cancer, but in their usual mode of use outside of an 'emergency' situation, these will not deliver the best long-term outcomes for patients as they have been surpassed and supplemented by other, intravenous, treatments.

A methodology that was stimulating interest prior to the COVID-19 pandemic but was utilised more widely during it (as a result of the promotion of oral agents) is metronomic chemotherapy treatment. Metronomic chemotherapy treatment refers to the chronic administration of low doses of chemotherapy that can sustain prolonged and active plasma levels of drugs, producing favourable tolerability in patients [11]. Many of the agents used in this technique are oral agents. Because of the high levels of tolerability, even in an older, frailer patient group, the use of metronomic chemotherapy has recently found favour in metastatic disease or employed later in lines of therapy. It has been found to be an effective option in breast and colorectal cancer [12]. During the COVID-19 pandemic, metronomic chemotherapy was employed relatively widely and found to be a reasonable option [12]. It is worth noting that metronomic chemotherapy is also of increased interest as a methodology to be employed in lower- and middle-income countries where oral agents, which can be more easily administered at home, combined with a more tolerable toxicity profile, could be of great help in delivering cancer care.

Another mode of delivering chemotherapy, and other SACT, is via the subcutaneous route. For similar reasons to the increased interest in oral SACT, the promotion of subcutaneous agents as possible alternatives to bringing patients in for IV treatments came to the fore, particularly during the early phase of the COVID-19 pandemic. As with oral agents, subcutaneous SACT has been used across Europe for many years. Subcutaneous agents that were widely employed prior to the COVID-19 pandemic include trastuzumab in breast cancer, bortezomib in haematological malignancy and rituximab in lymphoma. The use of rituximab has been linked with an increased level of hospitalisation and severity of infection in patients infected with SARS-CoV-2 [13] and so has fallen out of favour in recent years. Subcutaneous trastuzumab, however, was employed widely during the COVID-19 pandemic (either alone or in combination with pertuzumab) as was bortezomib. Even though subcutaneous agents reduce the need for extended stays in hospital in comparison to IV agents, there is still generally the need to have the drug administered by a trained healthcare professional, in most cases a nurse. Because of this, there was increased interest and trials of patients self-administering these agents during the COVID-19 pandemic, although in some cases this interest predated the COVID-19 pandemic [14]. Since 2020, there have been a number of trials of the self-administration of the biological agent bortezomib. Bortezomib is a targeted therapy used in the treatment of myeloma and is administered by subcutaneous injection. A team of researchers in Denmark [15] have shown that the self-administration of subcutaneous bortezomib in the homes of patients with myeloma was feasible and safe, saving patient and clinician time as well as reducing visits to hospital. During 2021 and 2022, the University College London Hospital launched a pilot bortezomib self-administration service [16] finding that administration could be safely delivered to improve overall patient experience and service efficiency. In further work carried out in the South East London Cancer Alliance, the number of subcutaneous agents self-administered by patients at home was expanded beyond bortezomib to include trastuzumab, cytarabine and denosumab [17]. The project reported that these agents had been successfully delivered via self-administration. The success was achieved via the production of pathway and governance policies, nurse training packages and drug-specific patient information leaflets. These were all put in place prior to implementation. It seems likely that the COVID-19 pandemic has driven a change which is likely to see a greater number of agents self-administered by patients in their own home with appropriate guidance and support.

Increased Deployment of Granulocyte-Colony-Stimulating Factor (GCSF)

Granulocyte-colony-stimulating factor (GCSF) is a growth factor that stimulates the bone marrow to produce granulocytes and stem cells and release them into the bloodstream. It has been known for some time that the use of GCSF alongside chemotherapeutic agents that cause bone marrow suppression will reduce the incidence of febrile neutropaenia and infection-related mortality [18]. Internationally, prior to the emergence of the COVID-19 pandemic, GCSF was typically used prophylactically in patients who had a greater than 20% risk of developing febrile neutropaenia [19]. During the COVID-19 pandemic, there was a general consensus to extend the use of GCSF to patients receiving SACT regimens where the risk of febrile neutropaenia was less than 20%, thereby administering GCSF to more patients receiving SACT [20]. In addition to this, despite there being little evidence to support the practice [21], some guidelines also recommended the use of GCSF to 'rescue' patients who developed febrile neutropaenia [22]. It should be noted that in the early days of the COVID-19 pandemic, there was concern that the use of GCSF may cause further harm in patients with active SARS-CoV-2 infection, due to its potential to augment the production of inflammatory cytokines. In practice there was little evidence that this represented a real risk. In terms of evaluation of the effectiveness of the increased use of GCSF during the COVID-19 pandemic and its role in maintaining patient safety, there is little evidence so far published that has considered this.

Vaccination and the Interplay with SACT Delivery

In December 2020, the United Kingdom became the first European country to licence a vaccine against the SARS-CoV-2 virus. This vaccine was produced by Pfizer/BioNTech, and two other vaccines shortly followed this, the Oxford/AstraZeneca vaccine and the Moderna vaccine, all of which were licensed and deployed across Europe in January 2021. Two of these vaccines (Pfizer/BioNTech and Moderna) utilise mRNA technology, and the third (Oxford/AstraZeneca) uses modified chimpanzee adenovirus as a vector.

In guidance first published in December 2020, the European Society of Medical Oncology pulled together the then-current guidance on patients with cancer and vaccination [23] resulting in a number of statements. These can be summarised as:

- People with cancer have an increased risk of severe COVID-19 and therefore should be vaccinated.
- Healthcare workers and other caregivers (e.g. family, caring for people with cancer) should be prioritised in receiving vaccination in order to minimise the chances of transmission.
- Close surveillance and monitoring of people with cancer are required after COVID-19 vaccination in order to assess potential adverse events and measure clinical outcomes.
- Physical distancing measures and other hygiene measures should accompany the optimisation of vaccination strategies.

When vaccinations first began to be deployed across Europe, there was uncertainty as to the effect these would have on patients receiving SACT. There was particular uncertainty around how patients receiving immunotherapy might react to the vaccines as both rely on stimulating an immune response. These concerns centred on whether the vaccines could reduce the efficacy of treatment or amplify side effects or adverse events. Fairly quickly evidence began to emerge that safety concerns were unlikely to be realised. Research from Israel in early 2021 showed that in 170 patients receiving immune checkpoint inhibitors, a similar rate of systemic adverse events after vaccination was experienced as those given more traditional chemotherapy [24] and that the vaccine side effect profile among the immunotherapy patients was generally comparable to that reported by a control group of age and sex-matched healthy individuals. Reassuringly a more recent meta-analysis published in 2023 [25] would seem to indicate that vaccination appears to be effective and safe in patients with cancer receiving immune checkpoint inhibitors.

At the time of writing, it is still difficult to assess the effect that vaccinations against the SARS-CoV-2 virus might have on the overall success of immunotherapy and clinical outcomes. What evidence there is would indicate that there may be some beneficial anti-cancer effects produced by being vaccinated whilst receiving immune checkpoint inhibitors, possibly via the activation of CD4 + T cells [26]. It should be stressed that the evidence is limited thus far to support this outside of narrow groups of patients with lung cancer.

An issue that led to some initial confusion and scheduling difficulties in SACT units and oncology clinics was the decision around the timing of vaccination for patients receiving SACT. The overall guidance across the United Kingdom and Europe was to complete vaccinating patients at least two weeks prior to commencing chemotherapy or SACT treatment. Where patients had already commenced treatment or required a vaccine booster, the advice was largely to vaccinate around two weeks prior to SACT delivery. The latest advice from the United Kingdom would indicate that this timing, although preferred, should be offset with the need to protect the patient from SARS-CoV-2 infection, also indicating that the evidence around the timing of vaccination was very limited [27].

Long-Term Impact of the COVID-19 Pandemic on SACT Delivery

In summary it can be stated that the short-term effects of the COVID-19 pandemic were largely negative with delays in treatment, disruption to standard treatments and high levels of patient distress.

It is also true that the need to protect patients, where the effects of SARS-CoV-2 infection in patients receiving treatment were largely unknown, accelerated changes to practice which were already in process. The move to telephone or 'virtual' SACT-related consultations is only partially tested in terms of effectiveness or patient experience but is now common practice and is unlikely to be rolled back. Increased use of GCSF during the pandemic has gone largely unevaluated but appears to have been effective in keeping patients out of hospital. The increased deployment of self-administration of subcutaneous agents has continued to be extended and widened, and this seems largely safe and effective. As time moves on, it may be easier to fully assess these changes.

Test Your Learning
1. What changes made to SACT delivery during the COVID-19 pandemic do you believe will remain in place and why?
2. How might we assess the overall effectiveness and tolerability of some of these changes?

References

1. Dai M, Liu D, Liu M, Zhou F, Li G, Chen Z et al (2020) Patients with cancer appear more vulnerable to SARS-COV-2: a multi-center study during the COVID-19 outbreak. Cancer Discov 10(6):83–791

2. Baxter MA, Murphy J, Cameron D et al (2021) The impact of COVID-19 on systemic anticancer treatment delivery in Scotland. Br J Cancer 124:1353–1356
3. Tan R et al (2022) Impact of immune checkpoint inhibitors on COVID-19 severity in patients with cancer. Oncologist 27(3):236–243
4. National Institute for Health and Care Excellence (NICE) (2020) Maintaining a cancer service in the midst of the COVID-19 pandemic: a single centre experience' NICE Shared Learning Database. Available at https://www.nice.org.uk/sharedlearning/maintaining-a-cancer-service-in-the-midst-of-the-covid-19-pandemic-a-single-centre-experience. Last Accessed Nov 2023
5. Muls A et al (2022) The psychosocial and emotional experiences of cancer patients during the COVID-19 pandemic: a systematic review. Semin Oncol (49) Issue 5:371–382
6. Miaskowski C et al (2021) Loneliness and symptom burden in oncology patients during the COVID-19 pandemic. Cancer 17(17):3246–3253
7. Macmillan Cancer Support (2020) The forgotten 'C'? : The impact of Covid-19 on cancer care. Macmillan cancer support. Available at https://www.macmillan.org.uk/_images/forgotten-c-impact-of-covid-19-on-cancer-care_tcm9-359174.pdf. Last Accessed Mar 2024
8. Watt et al (2020) Use of primary care during the COVID-19 pandemic. Published on-line by The Health Foundation. Available at https://www.health.org.uk/news-and-comment/charts-and-infographics/use-of-primary-care-during-the-covid-19-pandemic. Last Accessed Mar 2024
9. Camaniti C et al (2023) Psychosocial impact of virtual cancer care through technology: a systematic review and meta-analysis of randomized controlled trials. Cancers 15(7):2090
10. Shaffer KL et al (2023) Digital health and telehealth in cancer care: a scoping review of reviews. Lancet Digit Health 5:e316–e327
11. Cazzaniga ME, Cordani N, Capici S, Cogliati V, Riva F, Cerrito MG (2021) Metronomic chemotherapy. Cancers (Basel) 13(9):2236
12. Fedele P, Sanna V, Fancellu A, Marino A, Calvani N, Cinieri S (2021) De-escalating cancer treatments during COVID 19 pandemic: is metronomic chemotherapy a reasonable option? Crit Rev Oncol Hematol 157:103148
13. Varley CD, Winthrop KL (2021) Long-term safety of rituximab (risks of viral and opportunistic infections). Rheumatoid 23:74
14. Bittner B, Richter W, Schmidt J (2018) Subcutaneous Administration of Biotherapeutics: an overview of current challenges and opportunities. BioDrugs 32:425–440
15. Kirkegaard J et al (2022) Home is best. Self-administration of subcutaneous Bortezomib at home in patients with multiple myeloma – A mixed method study. European J Oncol Nursing 60:102199
16. Low M (2023) Assessment of the pilot bortezomib self-administration service at University College London NHS foundation trust (UCLH) a service audit. J Oncol Pharm Pract 29:15–16
17. So L, Davies LC, Oakley C, Shaunak N (2023) Patient self-administration of subcutaneous systemic anti-cancer therapy across South East London cancer Alliance (SELCA). J Oncol Pharm Pract 29:79–80
18. Kuderer NM, Dale DC, Crawford J, Lyman GH (2007) Impact of primary prophylaxis with granulocyte colony-stimulating factor on febrile neutropenia and mortality in adult cancer patients receiving chemotherapy: a systematic review. J Clin Oncol 2007(25):3158–3167
19. Klastersky J, de Naurois J, Rolston K (2016) Management of febrile neutropaenia: ESMO clinical practice guidelines. Ann Oncol 27(Suppl 5):v111–vv11
20. Aapro M et al (2021) (2021) - 'supportive care in patients with cancer during the COVID-19 pandemic'. ESMO Open 6(1):100038
21. NICE (2012) Neutropenic sepsis: prevention and management of neutropenic sepsis in cancer patients. Evidence review, search strategies, health economics evidence review and health economics plan: developed for NICE by the National Collaborating Centre for Cancer. UK NICE. Available at https://www.nice.org.uk/guidance/cg151/evidence/evidence-review-188303582. Last Accessed Feb 2024
22. American Society of Clinical Oncology (2020) 'COVID-19 patient care information. Available at: https://www.asco.org/asco-coronavirus-information/care-individuals-cancer-during-covid-19. Last Accessed Feb 2024

23. Castelo-Branco, L et al (2020) COVID-19 vaccination in cancer patients: ESMO statements
24. Waissengrin B et al (2021) Short-term safety of the BNT162b2 mRNA COVID-19 vaccine in patients with cancer treated with immune checkpoint inhibitors. Lancet Oncol; Published Online April 1, 2021, Available at https://www.thelancet.com/journals/lanonc/article/PIIS1470-2045(21)00155-8/fulltext. Last accessed Apr 2024
25. Ruiz JI et al (2023) COVID-19 vaccination in patients with cancer receiving immune checkpoint inhibitors: a systematic review and meta-analysis. J Immuno-Therapy Cancer 11:e006246
26. Qian Y, Zhu Z, Mo YY, Zhang Z (2023) COVID-19 vaccination is associated with enhanced efficacy of anti-PD-(L)1 immunotherapy in advanced NSCLC patients: a real-world study. Infect Agent Cancer 18(1):50
27. UK Health Security Agency (2023) COVID-19 vaccination programme: Information for healthcare practitioners' © Crown copyright 2023 Version 6.0. Available at https://assets.publishing.service.gov.uk/media/645a1ebe2226ee000c0ae432/COVID-19-vaccination-information-for-IHCP-v6.0-May2023.pdf. Last Accessed April 2024

Open Access This chapter is licensed under the terms of the Creative Commons Attribution 4.0 International License (http://creativecommons.org/licenses/by/4.0/), which permits use, sharing, adaptation, distribution and reproduction in any medium or format, as long as you give appropriate credit to the original author(s) and the source, provide a link to the Creative Commons license and indicate if changes were made.

The images or other third party material in this chapter are included in the chapter's Creative Commons license, unless indicated otherwise in a credit line to the material. If material is not included in the chapter's Creative Commons license and your intended use is not permitted by statutory regulation or exceeds the permitted use, you will need to obtain permission directly from the copyright holder.

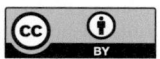

The Legacy of the COVID-19 Pandemic in Cancer Care

13

Helen Roe

Check Your Knowledge and Experience
1. Consider the impact the end of the pandemic had on both your ability to deliver care and importantly for patients receiving cancer care.
2. Recall the number of changes implemented during the pandemic that affected the delivery of cancer care. Consider how many are now 'standard' despite not having been evaluated.
3. Reflect on other world and UK events that have happened since the end of the pandemic in terms of everyday life and the delivery of cancer care.

Introduction

The COVID-19 pandemic had a huge impact on everyday living due to restrictions imposed by the governments of individual countries in an attempt to minimise the spread of the virus, reduce hospital admissions and the burden on healthcare. Day-to-day living was affected by the need for social distancing, the wearing of face coverings, staying at home and the need for mass vaccination programmes [1].

For patients with a cancer diagnosis, the implications were much greater as they were classed as being vulnerable due to their cancer diagnosis and potentially the treatment they were receiving. Many experienced delays in receiving necessary investigations, some had their treatment modified, and many experienced additional stresses as a consequence of the COVID-19 pandemic [2].

In the United Kingdom, even prior to the pandemic, there were issues with National Health Service (NHS) waiting times. It was generally felt that the demand for services had outstripped the available capacity, and this was evident by missed performance targets both in cancer care and beyond [3]. In 2023, a survey quantified

H. Roe (✉)
Northern Centre for Cancer Care (Cumbria) (up to Dec 2022),
Newcastle upon Tyne Hospitals NHS, Foundation Trust, Carlisle, UK

© The Author(s) 2026
M. Foulkes et al. (eds.), *Cancer Care in the Post-COVID World*,
https://doi.org/10.1007/978-3-031-33855-7_13

the negative impact these delays had on people's health and well-being; it found they had become increasingly lonely and suffered with increased anxiety and stress. Many people reported having appointments delayed or even cancelled [4]. Some of these routine appointments resulted in a delayed cancer diagnosis, especially if investigations were required, as up to 40% of cancer diagnoses result from routine diagnostics rather than specific cancer pathways [5].

During COVID Pandemic

Across the United Kingdom, there are specific cancer timeline standards and targets covering the pathway for a patient suspected of having cancer. Pre-pandemic the NHS cancer services had been under pressure, quantifiable by an inability to achieve these cancer waiting time targets [6].

The pandemic resulted in some of the repeated lowest performance figures regarding these targets, with fewer patients suspected of having cancer being referred from primary care organisations. The 62-day target (from urgent diagnosis to treatment) also generally demonstrated poor achievement figures although performance did improve between government-imposed 'lockdowns' [7].

A key factor in continued poor performance post pandemic and for waiting lists for cancer treatment continually growing is the shortage of key professionals across organisations. In England for June 2023, all four targets (urgent suspected cancer referral, 28-day faster diagnosis, the 62-day and 31-day decision to treatment) were all missed [6].

Healthcare services globally suffered the impact of the pandemic, resulting in interruptions to or modifications of normal care leading to an increased risk for patients with cancer [2]. Many changes were implemented based on minimal evidence and often on personal experience or recommendation. There was not the time to undertake audits or specific research prior to implementation.

There were many changes made to patient treatment including stopping neoadjuvant systemic anti-cancer treatment (SACT), halting adjuvant radiotherapy and commencing hormone treatment as an interim measure until surgery [8–11]. In the United Kingdom, a key priority was thorough documentation to ensure the individual plan could be revisited and evaluated as the COVID-19 pandemic progressed [12]. By revisiting and discussing the reasoning behind any changes, the patient and their family continued to be involved in the decision-making process regarding their care.

Chapter 4 described how technology was embraced as a way of communicating with patients and other professionals [2], and virtual reviews were implemented in many clinical settings [2, 8, 12, 13]. Certain investigations were also performed nearer to home with bloods and vital signs monitoring being undertaken by community healthcare teams. In light of these changes, some research protocols were amended accordingly. Patients reported toxicities and symptoms electronically in many cases but were still required to attend hospitals for imaging and other key investigations. The frequency of these tests was frequently reviewed and reduced [14].

Professionals found there to be an increase in patient engagement and satisfaction with virtual reviews leading to perceived improvements in the quality of care provided, and there was a drop in non-attendance for appointments making the clinics more cost-effective. The change to using telemedicine did require additional training for professionals, and in some cases, additional equipment required purchasing [12, 15]. However, questions continue to be raised regarding the number of remote consultations undertaken during the pandemic (via either video or telephone). In some cases, this may have resulted in poorer care and missed diagnosis due to the loss of direct observation or examination [5]. Some healthcare professionals perceived a lack of opportunity to observe nonverbal cues; however, even when patients did attend face-to-face consultations, face coverings were worn, again restricting the opportunity to observe facial expressions and some nonverbal cues [13]. In my own practice, one patient explained to me how she had learnt the importance of observing the eyes of the professional wearing a face covering as she gained much information from their eyes.

A pre-pandemic review of available evidence regarding the patients' experiences of teleconsultations in the surgical cancer setting in the United Kingdom found that they were widely acceptable in terms of convenience and saved money on transport and parking. The patients felt they received good service and that they had a sense of control during the consultation. However, they felt at times there was a lack of reassurance by not having a physical examination and missed the face-to-face support from professionals and other patients. They also missed the emotional support and nonverbal cues when telephone consultation took place. These findings reinforced the necessity for an appropriate mix of both face-to-face and virtual consultations dependent on the clinical situation [16].

Cancer research remains a vital service, and throughout the world, research activity was dramatically reduced and, in many cases, stopped due to the anticipated risk to cancer patients caused by the SARS-CoV-2 virus. [2, 14, 17] Patients also needed to adapt quickly during the pandemic in terms of symptom reporting as many paper questionnaires and face-to-face consultations were replaced by virtual symptom reporting using dedicated apps [14] and virtual appointments. These methodologies were being slowly introduced over the pre-pandemic years, but due to the COVID-19 pandemic, these became standard practice quickly for many people.

One example of how the pandemic necessitated a change in practice was previously a group of cancer patients meet face to face to receive health and well-being support sessions during their cancer journey. The pandemic caused this to stop, leaving them feeling isolated, lonely and unsure who to turn to for advice. The nursing team used digital technology to develop support via an online platform which the individual patient could access for personalised support at a time that was convenient for them. The platform utilised videos and podcasts as a way of sharing information and importantly had virtual cancer clinic workshops which allowed patients to meet face to face virtually. Continued patient feedback was paramount in the development and ongoing nature of this facility, which evaluated very well, and the patients felt better prepared and less anxious about the treatments they received. The team also offered a paper version depending on patient preference [18].

Following the COVID-19 Pandemic

Healthcare emerged from the COVID-19 pandemic and showed little resemblance to prior healthcare due to the implementation of required changes [2]. It was seen as a time to take stock of changes, their impact on patient care and clinical outcomes, plus initiate ways to evaluate the 'new norm', dispense with ineffective old practices and plan for the delivery of future healthcare across organisations [3, 7, 19].

Having experienced the pandemic, it became evident how healthcare providers struggled to provide specific care for patients with the SARS-CoV-2 virus and their specific needs, whilst they attempted to continue with all other care delivery. Despite cancer care being classed as a priority service, it became vital that resilience in the services was prioritised to assist the process of services 'bouncing back' to some kind of normality. To move forward the general public needed to have trust and confidence in their government and how the pandemic was managed. At times within the United Kingdom, this was lacking which may have led to an unwillingness to follow government rules and guidelines which had the aim of controlling the spread of the SARS-CoV-2 virus [19].

Shortly after the pandemic, towards the end of 2021, there were in excess of five and a half million people waiting for appointments, investigations and treatment within the NHS. The government allocated funding via the Elective Recovery Plan, which would provide additional checks and test, along with required treatments being delivered. However, for this to happen, there needed to be huge investment in the workforce to perform the required work and in IT provisions that were outdated and basic. It was also acknowledged that for changes to happen, developments needed to include all care providers working together and importantly that the focus should not be on numerical targets alone and should include a range of indicators depending on the services required [3].

Throughout the early part of the COVID-19 pandemic, the key message was to 'stay at home', and there was now a need through public health campaigns to encourage people to report symptoms and attend healthcare settings to have them investigated [5]. We witnessed the impact of the reduction in cancer screening due to attempts to reduce the risk of SARS-CoV-2 spreading, healthcare funding being relocated and a reduction in referral rates. This resulted in reductions in early cancer diagnosis for some people, i.e. those requiring a planned colonoscopy as part of their screening and ultimately led to delays in required surgery, both of which are associated with lower survival rates [1, 8, 20, 21]. To meet the demand and reduce the waiting lists, there would be a requirement for additional diagnostic capacity and closer collaboration between organisations and not merely a focus on cancer services [1, 5]. Already more flexible, working arrangements were introduced across organisations, for example, seven-day working and the introduction of diagnostic centres.

The COVID-19 pandemic exacerbated the continued failure to meet key cancer standards as concerns escalated regarding recruiting and importantly retaining professionals to deliver the care as every failed target resulted in a patient being kept waiting for treatment and increasingly waiting for longer [6]. There was a need to review service provision both in primary and secondary organisations in an attempt to capture all possible patients and reduce the overwhelming backlog of patients requiring diagnostic interventions as part of their potential cancer pathway [7, 22].

In Canada, modelling to assess the future impact of the various delays due to the pandemic demonstrated an increase in late-stage cancer diagnoses and mortality. As we have seen, the COVID-19 pandemic led to patient delays in seeking advice, delays in screening and diagnostics to reach a diagnosis and delays in patients receiving treatment. All these scenarios left patients potentially at risk of delayed diagnosis, developing more advanced disease at presentation and, for some, increased mortality [21].

Where changes necessitated during the COVID-19 pandemic have continued, there is a clear need for them to be evaluated and recognised as standard care or to revert to original ones if indicated [14]. There is also a need for specific research to be undertaken to establish how patients access services and support as part of their daily lives that changed greatly due to the pandemic [22]. Some changes remaining in practice could result in cost reductions or be time-saving in connection with clinical staff commitments. Other benefits may be greater collaboration across pathways by bringing together different clinical teams and not only focusing on the oncology team [14].

Following the pandemic would have been the ideal opportunity to assess for resilience in healthcare services, be proactive in developing services for any future event, whether planned or unforeseen like the pandemic [15, 19, 22]. However, no sooner were pandemic restrictions reduced or removed, then people started feeling the impact of the cost-of-living crisis, the war in Ukraine and the impact of striking healthcare workers. All these events have had a negative impact on healthcare delivery and led to increased waiting lists and delays in diagnosis and initiating planned treatments.

Throughout the pandemic, many healthcare professionals worked additional hours to ensure patients received required care, at times in unfamiliar working environments. On occasion, they put themselves at potentially greater risk of infection due to their patient-facing roles combined with variable access to personal protective equipment [12, 23]. Professionals who previously coped with their everyday work may have struggled during the COVID-19 pandemic, and for many, their mental health was affected, largely due to the many uncertainties around COVID and the future [24]. Some displayed signs of stress, anxiety, depression, sleeplessness and in some cases even contemplated taking their own life [23]. Other impacts of the pandemic on professionals' well-being ultimately resulted in negative consequences on their work, home life and importantly the care they provided. There were often conversations around what was classed as appropriate screening and which professional groups were able to access COVID testing kits. A key factor for some professional groups was that a positive COVID test meant that they were not able to continue to work in their clinical areas for a period. If they had a job that did not facilitate them working from home, this left a feeling of failure as they considered the negative impact this could have on their colleagues from a staffing point of view.

The European Society for Medical Oncology (ESMO), through a global survey, demonstrated the impact the pandemic had caused especially in terms of increased levels of distress and burnout. Professionals felt there was a clear need to implement measures to improve present and future resilience in services as well as addressing professional well-being [25]. Despite the impact on their personal lives and potentially that of their families, they remained focused on delivering patient care [26]. Similarly, a cross-sectional, multinational study undertaken during the pandemic showed significant levels of burnout, diminished coping abilities and reduced resilience amongst cancer care professionals [27]. ESMO Resilience Taskforce following their survey highlighted the consequences of the pandemic on professionals and developed support solutions for both organisations and individuals around topics such as working hours, the impact of the pandemic on training and clinical research and improving staff resilience to change in the future [25].

In the United Kingdom, the pandemic affected the mental well-being of professionals by increasing their workload, by redeployment to unfamiliar working environment and an expectation to work longer hours [24], causing concerns for their and their family's health [12] as well as the emotional impact of seeing the number of patients die. In addition, there was an overwhelming concern regarding the standard of care they could provide. These concerns often resulted in them demonstrating signs of depression, anxiety, stress, burnout and other mental health conditions [23, 26]. Any resulting time off work exacerbated the pressure on colleagues. The professional consequences of the pandemic seen in the United Kingdom therefore mirrored the findings of surveys undertaken by ESMO [25].

From my own practice, I can recall one nurse who worked as part of the chemotherapy team who moved out of her family home into provided accommodation to minimise her risk of acquiring COVID or placing her family at risk due to continuing in her role. We were all part of a 'work bubble', which impacted our everyday living throughout the pandemic, and even when the government reduced the restrictions on the general public, we continued in our bubble for longer to safeguard the patients requiring SACT and in an attempt to maintain our workforce at a safe level. At times colleagues describe how they felt isolated and generally lacked support, describing how acknowledgement, not necessarily praise, would have provided a boost to their morale.

Professionals caring for patients with cancer were already at a higher risk of burnout and exhaustion due to the nature of a cancer diagnosis in terms of the psychological impact, caring for both the patient and their family along with their everyday professional responsibilities [27]. As we have seen in Chap. 8 on the psychological impact of the COVID-19 pandemic, an important requirement in supporting professionals effectively was access to a supportive manager in whom they could discuss any concerns, which could have impacted their mental health [24]. From the experience of colleagues, this was something that many felt they lacked, which could have been due to the many changing priorities the NHS was facing.

A survey on the effect of the COVID-19 pandemic undertaken by ESMO demonstrated that healthcare professionals still faced increased demands on both their role and them as individuals. This was largely due to the continued redeployment of professionals and a deterioration in working conditions. This led to difficulties in delivering care at a standard they wished to. Combined with the reduction in clinical trial activities, alterations to standard SACT options and a reduction in cancer screening investigations left professionals concerned regarding the long-term negative impact of the COVID-19 pandemic on patients with cancer [12, 28].

Throughout the COVID-19 pandemic, it became evident that there was a decline in professionals' satisfaction with the quality of care they were able to provide. An annual survey undertaken late in 2022 demonstrated a drop in the number of nurses who were happy with the standard of care provided by their organisation. They largely attributed this to staff shortages impacting on clinical effectiveness. Some described an increase in clinical errors they had experienced and near misses that could have consequences for patients or professionals. Many felt under increased pressure whilst at work and felt that their individual mental health and general well-being were adversely affected. The results of this survey demonstrated how nurses felt staffing levels were affecting both staff morale and patients. In the United Kingdom at this time, there was also nursing dissatisfaction with their current pay [29].

To compound this, another survey from the United Kingdom in 2022 demonstrated how dissatisfied junior doctors were with their working conditions and pay with many planning to leave the NHS for another job or planned to work abroad [30, 31].

Ongoing surveys undertaken by ESMO demonstrated that professionals continued to feel overwhelmed by the pressure they were placed under, citing concerns regarding their individual safety at work as COVID-19 figures remained high. They also commented that their personal/family time had reduced, and many reported not being able to take time off for annual leave and/or study leave. The figures relating to individual well-being were worse, and the risk of burnout had increased, with around one in four professionals considering changing their career, including leaving oncology, due to perceiving a decline in support [28]. These issues were referred to as arising post pandemic, but staffing shortages, funding issues and low staff morale were all known about pre-pandemic [26].

In the United Kingdom, the growing unrest amongst healthcare professionals regarding their pay and working conditions reached a pivotal moment when professionals felt their only option to be heard was to take industrial action. They were not the only groups reaching this decision as the education and transport sectors also chose to take industrial action. By July 2023 nurses, doctors, dentists, radiographers, ambulance services and paramedics had all carried out industrial action. One report documented that one 28-hour strike by nurses resulted in 7600 cancellations in acute care. July 2023 saw the eighth month of industrial action in the United Kingdom, and despite professionals continuing to provide the most urgent care, this action ultimately did impact patients due to over 365,000 staff absent and around 600,000 cancelled appointments by this month [32].

By late 2023 in the NHS, some professional groups accepted the pay offers made by the government and returned to previous working patterns, but medical staff continued to take strike action, meaning continued disruption for patients and the NHS's ability to reduce the long waiting lists. At the time of writing, in late 2023, this industrial action has continued to have a major impact on patients with around 900,00 rescheduled appointments and procedures [33], and this figure will continue to increase until agreement is reached between the UK government and the unions.

The European Cost of Living Crisis

Across Europe in the post-COVID-19 period during 2021, food and energy cost had continued to rise, especially fuel prices. Many of these rises were because of the COVID-19 pandemic which were later exacerbated by the conflict in Ukraine. Along with the general population, healthcare professionals were also experiencing the impact of the cost-of-living crisis, having to cut back buying food and heating their homes to make ends meet [31, 34].

For patients with cancer, the consequences of the cost-of-living crisis had a far greater impact as many had already received a diagnosis and started delayed treatment and were incurring out-of-pocket expenses relating to their cancer diagnosis [35]. In the United Kingdom, one charity described how many cancer patients were potentially putting their health at risk by the choices they needed to make and that nearly a quarter of cancer patients were either buying less food or making fewer hot meals to cut costs. These figures included patients who were receiving treatment. Due to the increase in energy and other household bills, around one million cancer patients in the United Kingdom who responded to a survey were making the decision to wear additional layers of clothing in their homes to stay warm and save on heating costs. Another way they saved money was to wash clothes and bedding less frequently [28, 35].

The impact of the weak economy which followed the COVID-19 pandemic was evident. There was evidence of reduced treatment adherence, especially amongst vulnerable groups. Concerns were raised regarding the mental health of individuals and its impact on making decisions including medication adherence [36]. Professionals needed to be aware of this potential impact on patients with cancer when they prioritised their spendings professionals increasingly needed to consider the patients' ability to pay for the out-of-pocket costs they incurred as part of their treatment, for example, supportive medication bought over the counter and travel costs [35, 36].

Further research revealed that around a quarter of cancer patients were concerned about the impact the cost-of-living crisis would have on them and over three-quarters felt it was affecting their prognosis. Some patients were so concerned about their financial requirements they chose to return to work sooner than planned. Half felt they would struggle to pay for food, and two-thirds felt they would struggle with their heating bills [37]. One key area of concern related to cost incurred by attending hospital appointments but given the adoption of telemedicine during the pandemic which continued they only needed to attend hospitals, when necessary, rather than as a routine.

Professionals had an increased requirement to assess each patient individually and signpost them to local or national charities for psychological and potential financial support and/or refer them to government services regarding benefits they may be entitled to claim, especially if not working due to their diagnosis and/or treatment they were receiving.

Opportunities to Prepare and Move Forward

The post-COVID-19 pandemic period provided an opportunity to learn from the experience of the pandemic and prepare future services to deliver equitable cancer care to all who need it irrespective of individual circumstances or global events [22]. The opportunity exists to promote both a proactive and a reactive approach to innovation and resilience in times of humanitarian crises, such as a pandemic. In healthcare, improved resilience should result in the development of new goals and importantly building a coordinated response should such an event happen again [3, 19].

As we have learnt, due to the potential number of late cancer diagnoses as well as an aging population, health provision across Europe needs to be able to accommodate an increased demand on diagnostic services, surgical provision and treatment opportunities, all of which will require investment and a major overall of current services [22]. Much can be learnt from studies undertaken during the pandemic which explored the services from the prospective of the patient which will support future developments. One such study explored cancer patients' decision-making process regarding accessing clinical trials balanced with their fears relating to the need for social distancing and possibly contracting COVID [38].

The pandemic resulted in many delays for patients which has now formed a huge 'backlog'. The challenge of clearing these backlogs that were present at the end of the pandemic has placed a massive challenge on healthcare professionals who had given so much during the pandemic and now faced another huge challenge [3, 12]. This situation must be viewed as an opportunity to review and change outdated practices and work closer with colleagues to ensure going forward that models of care delivery were safe and effective for all [3, 22].

Due to delays in appointments, investigations, receiving a diagnosis and commencing treatment caused by the pandemic the impact will continue for many years [1, 5, 21]. One challenge will be the pressure on key diagnostic services such as radiology and pathology which were greatly impacted by the demands of COVID-19 screening [8, 22]. Newly diagnosed patients require prompt diagnostics and a diagnosis, prior to commencing required treatment. Their needs will require balancing against existing patients who will require a full clinical review in terms of possible changes in original treatment plan and treatment received, which may have changed during the pandemic possible changes in their initial prognosis, not to mention non-cancer patient's needs. Changes will only enhance patient care and reduce longer waiting times if there is a review of existing diagnostic services, greater use of new innovations and increased use of technology such as remote consultations and artificial intelligence (AI), along with staffing reviews, all of which will require investment [15].

Other innovations implemented during the pandemic included virtual multidisciplinary team meetings, remote working, home delivery of medicines or 'drive-through' facilities, SACT at home and a greater use of local community services [39]. These should now be reviewed from both a patient and professional perspective and evidence-based decisions made to evaluate if they should continue in post-COVID-19 pandemic practice. The rapid adoption of remote working early in the pandemic was not without many logistical challenges for some [24] and with the need for professionals to return to clinical areas, meaning the time is right to review when remote working benefits both the patient and professional.

Throughout the pandemic there was a need for clear documentation for each individual patient which would have been evaluated on a regular basis. Now following the pandemic, the importance of this documentation should also be utilised in terms of establishing the current situation, assessing the impact of the pandemic on risk stratification of specific cancers and comorbidities, along with planning resources to manage the backlog and future demands on services [12]. All professionals must have an active role in identifying and monitoring overdue investigations and, for those receiving treatments, assessing clinical outcomes and determining individual care plans for patients [21]. It is vital all patients undergo a clinical review as some guidance has been removed post pandemic [9].

When considering the impact of the pandemic on professionals, one key learning should be around the provision of staff psychological support, especially as the long-term effects on them is unknown and many are demonstrating psychological effects. Many professionals were so focused on patients and delivering care they at times inadvertently neglected their own health and well-being, even though for some their experience of the pandemic could be described as resembling a trauma [12]. Organisations need to acknowledge the impact of the pandemic on all employees and implement processes which focus on the mental health and well-being of their employees by providing training for them focused on identifying possible signs of psychological distress in themselves and in others. Mental health needs to be a subject that is openly discussed and not seen as a weakness, one which allows professionals to share experiences and speak openly, collectively or if they wish to have private individual discussions [23, 24].

Services should be in place which professionals feel able to access to discuss their individual feelings and mental health issues and having confidence that they will not experience negative repercussions in the workplace. There has been an increase in such services which have been openly accessed by various professional groups, and these are also seen as a way of acknowledging the impact the pandemic had on individuals and that lessons are being learnt [26].

Conclusion

In summary the consequences of the COVID-19 pandemic were not all negative and had provided the opportunity for positive transformation in terms of service delivery. The use of virtual healthcare has impacted service capacity and provided cost savings for many patients. Virtual education and support resulted in time savings for many and offered the opportunity for greater numbers to participate. There has been evidence of greater access to clinical trials due to changes implemented during the pandemic, removing the need for some face-to-face consultations, and in the way, consent is provided and data collection throughout a trial [17]. The greater use of electronic signatures has been seen as a huge improvement across all aspects of services from signing consultation letters, prescribing and confirming results of investigations. With most of this taking place electronically, this offers greater opportunities for monitoring and less paperwork. The development of online platforms offering patient support via podcasts, videos and virtual cancer clinics is an initiative that could be adapted to meet local service needs across the world to better support patients and provide an alternative to hospital attendance [18].

The NHS in England recognised the vital contribution of professionals and acknowledged that the workforce overall had not previously been planned in a coordinated manner. This meant that the best use of professional skills had been limited, forecasting for future needs of services and a need to act on them in a timely way. The impact of the pandemic had been a challenge for the NHS due to the new demands it placed on the services and on professionals. They concluded that now was the time to review the NHS and that this would be achieved through the Long-Term Workforce Plan. The plan aims to highlight shortfalls, developing strategies to correct them and importantly the commitment of investment to undertake them. They acknowledged one area requiring urgent action remains its workforce and the need for growth in line with demands. They will incorporate required education across all professional groups and ensuring professionals function to their full potential by expanding advanced practice training and new ways of recruiting and retaining professionals. Another key area of the plan which will have a major impact on healthcare is the embracement of newer developments to assist professionals to prevent diseases, diagnose, treat and manage them when they occur. Moving forward a key focus is to be on the individual patient through personalised care out of the hospital setting [15].

During the COVID-19 pandemic, there was renewed interest in the use of AI in healthcare. AI has the potential to impact both patient outcomes and demand on the service [15]. AI has shown to have a place in mammography screening, and clinical safety analysis has been performed during the Mammography Screening with Artificial Intelligence (MASAI) trial. Retrospective studies in Sweden have shown promising results when the use of AI was used to improve mammography screening whilst also reducing the amount of professionals' time reading mammograms [40]. Routine mammography for low-risk patients results in a small proportion of breast cancer detection yet generates large numbers of mammograms which require reading by radiologists [41]. Results of the MASAI trial demonstrated a similar rate of cancer detection for mammograms reported using AI as for those which had undergone double reading by radiologists and importantly reduced their workload in relation to routine mammography screening, annual screening for moderate hereditary risk or a history of breast cancer [40]. An AI-based mammography screening protocol for breast cancer was developed with strict criteria in terms of individual risk groups. This demonstrated that the workload of the radiologists could be greatly reduced, and the number of false positives also reduced. Similar practice changes have been reported from other countries and have shown that appropriate use of AI reporting is a way to safely reduce the radiologist's workload and potentially improving patient screening outcomes and does warrant further exploration [41].

Another area in cancer care where AI has a place is the planning process for radiotherapy, especially for lung, prostate and colorectal cancers. During the summer of 2023, the National Institute for Health and Care Excellence (NICE) in the United Kingdom published draft guidance for consideration. AI has the potential to save both professionals' time and costs, whilst not compromising patient care. AI would be used during planning (contouring) to ensure the treatment targets the cancer and avoids surrounding healthy cells and organs which is currently performed by a radiographer. The final images would still require reviewing by the healthcare professional, but the time saved would enable more face-to-face contact with a patient in terms of support and reduce the current treatment waiting lists [42].

It is also envisaged that virtual consultations will continue in future service delivery, even though face-to-face consultation has slowly been reintroduced following the pandemic. Considerations will need to be given to which appointment type is correct for the individual patient and the situation, i.e. follow-up on treatment, needed to discuss clinical changes or a need for examination [12, 16].

The COVID-19 pandemic has changed cancer care for all, from the patients receiving the care, families supporting them and the professionals delivering it. By taking the positives from changes implemented along the way, service pathways can be reviewed and developed to be more supportive of individual patients' specific needs. There is a need to build on future development of psychological services alongside newer developments in treatment options, aided by continued research into all aspects of care. Professionals require changes in their current working practices in terms of workload, education and psychological support to continue to function effectively and meet patient demand, which will only continue to increase until the backlogs are reduced [15, 22]. Finally, professionals need to feel valued for their contribution by colleagues and not just be the patients they care for. The future of cancer care will be challenging but ultimately rewarding.

In the final analysis, it might be that the lasting legacy of the COVID-19 pandemic on cancer care will not be the impact on cancer survival, incidence or management but on the psychological effect it has had on those working in cancer care and on the shaken belief within the European populations that modern healthcare can continue to be delivered seamlessly no matter what the circumstance. It is imperative that the mental well-being of the cancer workforce is addressed and also that robust plans are put in place to address future pandemics based on the learning from the collective recent experience.

Conflict of Interest The Author does not have any conflict of interest to declare.

References

1. Rucinska M, Nawrocki S (2022) COVID-19 pandemic: Impact on cancer patients. Int J Environ Res Public Health. https://www.ncbi.nlm.nih.gov/pmc/articles/PMC9564768/pdf/ijerph-19-12470.pdf. Accessed Feb 2024
2. Jazieh A et al (2020) Impact of the COVID-19 pandemic on cancer care: a global collaborative study. J Clin Oncol (Global Oncology) 6:1428–1438. https://ascopubs.org/doi/pdf/10.1200/GO.20.00351?role=tab. Accessed February 2024
3. House of Commons Health + Social Care Committee (2021) Clearing the backlog caused by the pandemic. https://committees.parliament.uk/publications/8352/documents/85020/default/. Accessed Feb 2024
4. Office for National Statistics (2023) Tracking the impact of winter pressures in Great Britain: November 2022–February 2023. https://www.ons.gov.uk/peoplepopulationandcommunity/wellbeing/articles/trackingtheimpactofwinterpressuresingreatbritain/november2022tofebruary2023. Accessed Feb 2024
5. Maringe C et al (2020) The impact of the COVID-19 pandemic on cancer deaths due to delay in diagnosis in England, UK: a national, population-based, modelling study. Lancet 21. https://www.thelancet.com/action/showPdf?pii=S1470-2045%2820%2930388-0. Accessed February 2024
6. Lowes S (2023) Cancer waiting times latest updates and analysis. https://news.cancerresearchuk.org/2023/09/14/cancer-waiting-times-latest-updates-and-analysis/. Accessed Sep 2023
7. Fox L et al (2021) Association between COVID-19 burden and delays to diagnosis and treatment of cancer patients in England. J Cancer Policy. https://www.ncbi.nlm.nih.gov/pmc/articles/PMC8653402/pdf/main.pdf. Accessed Feb 2024
8. Richards M et al (2020) The impact of the COVID-19 pandemic on cancer care. Nature Cancer 1:565–567. https://www.nature.com/articles/s43018-020-0074-y. Accessed Feb 2024
9. National Institute for Health and Care Excellence (NICE) (2020) COVID-19 rapid guideline: delivery of systemic anticancer treatments. https://www.nice.org.uk/guidance/ng161/resources/covid19-rapid-guideline-delivery-of-systemic-anticancer-treatments-pdf-66141895710661. Accessed Aug 2023
10. NHS (2021) NHS England interim treatment options during the COVID-19 pandemic. https://www.theacp.org.uk/userfiles/file/resources/covid_19_resources/nhs-england-interim-treatment-options-during-the-covid19-pandemic-pdf-8715724381-6-jan-2021.pdf. Accessed Feb 2024
11. National Cancer Drug Fund (CDF) (2022) National Cancer Drugs Fund List V1.231 -Section C. Interim systemic anti-cancer therapy (SACT) treatment change options during the COVID-19 pandemic. https://www.england.nhs.uk/wp-content/uploads/2017/04/national-cdf-list-v1.231.pdf. Accessed March 2023
12. Tsang-Wright F et al (2020) Breast cancer surgery after the COVID-19 pandemic. Future Oncol 16(33):2687–2690. https://www.futuremedicine.com/doi/epub/10.2217/fon-2020-0619. Accessed February 2024
13. Dhada S et al (2021) Cancer Service during the COVID-19 pandemic: systematic review of patient's and caregiver's experiences. Cancer Manag Res 13:5875–5887. https://www.ncbi.nlm.nih.gov/pmc/articles/pmid/34349561/. Accessed Feb 2024
14. Morton C et al (2023) Revitalising cancer trials post pandemic: time for reform. Br J Cancer 128:1409–1414. https://www.ncbi.nlm.nih.gov/pmc/articles/PMC10035974/pdf/41416_2023_Article_2224.pdf. Accessed Feb 2024
15. NHS England (2023) NHS Long Term Workforce Plan. https://www.england.nhs.uk/wp-content/uploads/2023/06/nhs-long-term-workforce-plan-v1.2.pdf. Accessed Feb 2024

16. Francheska B et al (2023) Patients' experience of teleconsultations in the UK. Br J Nurs 32(10):S24–S29. https://www.britishjournalofnursing.com/content/remote-follow-up/patients-experience-of-teleconsultations-in-the-uk/. Accessed Feb 2024
17. Buckley-Mellor O (2020) What's happened to cancer clinical trials during the COVID-19 pandemic? https://news.cancerresearchuk.org/2020/11/04/whats-happened-to-cancer-clinical-trials-during-the-covid-19-pandemic/. Accessed Feb 2024
18. Tweddie C (2023) Digital health post pandemic: turning quick fixes into long-term improvements. Br J Nurs 32(17):S26–S27. https://www.britishjournalofnursing.com/content/bjn-awards/digital-health-post-pandemic-turning-quick-fixes-into-long-term-improvements. Accessed Sep 2023
19. Sagan A et al (2023) Assessing resilience of a health system is difficult but necessary to prepare for the next crisis. Br Med J. https://www.bmj.com/content/bmj/382/bmj-2022-073721.full.pdf. Accessed Jan 2024
20. Mazidimoradi A, Tiznobaik A, Salehiniya H (2022) impact of the COVID-19 pandemic on colorectal cancer screening: a systematic review. Journal of Gastrointestinal. Cancer 53:730–744. https://www.ncbi.nlm.nih.gov/pmc/articles/PMC8371036/pdf/12029_2021_Article_679.pdf. Accessed Jan 2024
21. Wilkinson A (2022) Mitigating COVID-19's impact on missed and delayed cancer diagnoses. Can Fam Physician 68. https://www.ncbi.nlm.nih.gov/pmc/articles/PMC9097737/pdf/0680323.pdf. Accessed Jan 2024
22. Cancer Research UK (2022) Impact of the COVID-19 pandemic on cancer surgery and cancer mortality. https://telstrahealth.co.uk/wp-content/uploads/2022/09/Telstra-Health-UK-CRUK-report.pdf. Accessed Jan 2024
23. Shah M et al (2021) Mental health and COVID-19: The psychological implications of a pandemic for nurses. Clin J Oncol Nurs 25(1):P69–P75. https://doi.org/10.1188/21.CJON.69-75. https://www.ons.org/cjon/25/1/mental-health-and-covid-19-psychological-implications-pandemic-nurses. Accessed Jan 2024
24. Greenberg N et al (2020) How might the NHS protect the mental health of health-care workers after the COVID-19 crisis? Lancet 7. https://www.thelancet.com/action/showPdf?pii=S2215-0366%2820%2930224-8. Accessed Jan 2024
25. Banerjee S et al (2021) The impact of COVID-19 on oncology professionals: results of the ESMO Resilience Task Force survey collaboration. https://www.ncbi.nlm.nih.gov/articles/pmid/33601295/. Accessed Jan 2024
26. House of Commons Health & Social Care Committee (2021) Workforce burnout and resilience on the NHS and Social Care. https://committees.parliament.uk/publications/6158/documents/68766/default/. Accessed Feb 2024
27. Cloconi C, Economou M, Charalambous A (2023) Burnout, coping and resilience of the cancer care workforce during the SARS-CoV-2: A multinational cross-sectional study. Eur J Oncol Nurs 63. https://doi.org/10.1016/j.ejon.2022.102204. http://hdl.handle.net/20.500.14279.29633. Accessed Dec 2023
28. Lim K et al (2021) The impact of COVID-19 on oncology professionals- one year on: lessons learned from the ESMO Resilience Task Force survey series. https://www.ncbi.nlm.nih.gov/pmc/articles/pmid/35007996/. Accessed Feb 2024
29. Royal College of Nursing (2023) NHS England survey 'lays bare' staff in crisis, says RCN, warning change cannot wait. www.rcn.org.uk/news-and-events/Press-Release/nhs-staff-survey. Accessed Dec 2023
30. Ratwatte M (2023) The NHS workforce crisis is a retention crisis. Br Med J 380:602. https://www.bmj.com/content/380/bmj.p602.full.print. Accessed Feb 2024
31. Waters A (2022) A third of junior doctors plan to leave NHS to work abroad in next 12 months. https://doi.org/10.1136/bmj.o3066. Accessed February 2024
32. NHS England (2023) Information for the public on industrial action. https://www.england.nhs.uk/long-read/information-for-the-public-on-industrial-action/. Accessed Feb 2024
33. Department of Health and Social Care & Steve Barclay MP (2023) Government considers minimum service levels in hospitals during strikes. https://www.gov.uk/government/

news/government-considers-minimum-service-levels-in-hospitals-during-strikes. Accessed Feb 2024
34. Office for National Statistics (2023) Cost of living latest insights. https://www.ons.gov.uk/economy/inflationandpriceindices/articles/costofliving/latestinsights. Accessed Dec 2023
35. Lancet Oncology (2022) Cancer, health-care backlogs, and the cost of living crisis. Lancetcom Oncol 23:691. https://www.thelancet.com/action/showPdf?pii=S1470-2045%2822%2900302-3. Accessed Feb 2024
36. Agh T, van Boven J, Kardas P (2023) Europe's cost of living crisis jeopardises medication adherence. Br Med J 380:747. https://doi.org/10.1136/bmj.p747. Accessed Feb 2024
37. Maggie's (2022) People with cancer more worried about cost of living than diagnosis. https://www.maggies.org/about-us/news/people-with-cancer-more-worried-about-cost-of-living-than-diagnosis/. Accessed Feb 2024
38. Hood B (2023) Understanding the experiences of cancer patients referred for a clinical trial during the COVID-19 pandemic. British J Nursing 32(2):82–87. https://doi.org/10.12968/bjon.2023.32.2.82. Accessed Feb 2024
39. Cancer Research UK (2021) COVID innovations in cancer treatment. https://www.cancerresearchuk.org/sites/default/files/covid_innovations_-_treatment_1.pdf. Accessed Feb 2024
40. Lang K et al (2023) Artificial intelligence-supported screen reading versus standard double reading in the mammography screening with artificial intelligence trial (MASAI): a clinical safety analysis of a randomised, controlled, non-inferiority, single-blinded, screening accuracy study. Lancet 22(8):936–944. https://www.thelancet.com/journals/lanonc/article/PIIS1470-2045(23)00298-X/fulltext. Accessed Feb 2024
41. Lauritzen A et al (2022) An artificial intelligence-based mammography screening protocol for breast cancer: Outcome and Radiology Workload. Radiology 304:41–49. https://pubs.rsna.org/doi/epdf/10.1148/radiol.210948. Accessed February 2024
42. National Institute for Health & Social Care (NICE) (2023) Artificial intelligence technologies to speed up contouring in radiotherapy treatment planning. https://www.nice.org.uk/news/article/artificial-intelligence-technologies-to-speed-up-contouring-in-radiotherapy-treatment-planning. Accessed Feb 2024

Open Access This chapter is licensed under the terms of the Creative Commons Attribution 4.0 International License (http://creativecommons.org/licenses/by/4.0/), which permits use, sharing, adaptation, distribution and reproduction in any medium or format, as long as you give appropriate credit to the original author(s) and the source, provide a link to the Creative Commons license and indicate if changes were made.

The images or other third party material in this chapter are included in the chapter's Creative Commons license, unless indicated otherwise in a credit line to the material. If material is not included in the chapter's Creative Commons license and your intended use is not permitted by statutory regulation or exceeds the permitted use, you will need to obtain permission directly from the copyright holder.

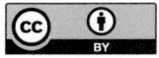

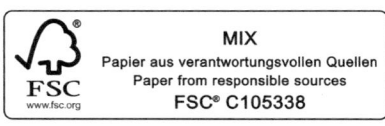

If you have any concerns about our products,
you can contact us on
ProductSafety@springernature.com

In case Publisher is established outside the EU,
the EU authorized representative is:
**Springer Nature Customer Service Center GmbH
Europaplatz 3, 69115 Heidelberg, Germany**

Printed by Libri Plureos GmbH
in Hamburg, Germany